The Weight Issue

- it's your genes plus modern living

How to make an individual weight loss plan based on
medical evidence

Dr A. E. Oates

CONTENTS

Introduction

Why should you read this book?

Although there are many books available aimed at helping with weight loss, this book is different. It takes a new look at the whole issue of excess weight, based on the available medical evidence. It will help you to work out the cause of your weight problem and to make an individual plan to lose excess weight.

I have a medical degree and have worked in general practice and other specialties, so I have been able to review the research surrounding the subject. Some of the evidence regarding the cause and management of weight gain is not widely known among the medical profession, let alone the general public. This book hopes to dispel some of the myths associated with excess weight. Certainly, my own attitudes have changed since researching this book. I used to think the solution to a weight problem was to "eat less and exercise more" whereas now my first thought is more likely to be, "it's their genes".

This book will answer the following questions:

- What is the cause of your weight problem?
- Will having excess weight affect your health?
- Which diets work? What is the evidence from medical trials of various diets?
- Will exercise work for you? (It doesn't help everyone with weight loss.)
- How should you cope with the stigma that goes with excess weight?
- What should you actually do to lose weight and keep it off?

If you are overweight, it is not your fault but is due to your inherited genes combined with other factors. The tendency to eat automatically, "comfort" eating and the changes in modern food availability, can all contribute to a weight problem. Most people are unaware that weight is inherited to the same extent that height is inherited. There is no need to attach blame to the problem. Those people who lose weight and successfully keep the weight off for a period of years, do so by following an individual plan. This book gives the scientific evidence that can help you to lose excess weight and more importantly, prevent weight regain.

If having extra weight is not your fault, then why worry about it? Unless you are particularly vain, you will want to know whether there is likely to be an effect on your health. The statistics concerning the effect of weight are clear. Being overweight or mildly obese is not likely to increase the chance of early death, and the association of weight with illness is put into perspective in Chapter 2. It has been found that larger people are often treated disrespectfully by the medical profession (they are the most common targets for derogatory humour from doctors) and you will also find strategies for dealing with this sort of discrimination in this book.

You will want to know whether diets "work" and the medical evidence for their effectiveness. Chapter 3 looks at various diets, including the popular "intermittent fasting" diet, diets which vary proportions of fat, protein and carbohydrates, glycemic index diet, very low calorie diets (such as followed by Oprah years ago), commercial diets, meal replacements (such as Slim Fast), pre-packaged meals (such as Jenny Craig) and diet websites. Most diets cause weight loss in the first six months and this is often followed by partial or total regain. Long term success hinges on finding something that works for the individual, and this book aims to help the reader to find a regime that will work for them personally.

It is a myth that exercise always helps with weight loss. In fact, some of us will lose weight with exercise, but others compensate by eating more. Chapter 4 will help you to decide which category you fall into. Gender and age can make a difference. Men tend to lose weight with exercise and women get less relative benefit.

Preventing weight regain is more difficult than losing it in the first place. Chapter 5 discusses the evidence that some strategies to avoid weight regain are much more successful than others. The sort of eating regime you have, the frequency of weight monitoring, and even the way in which you think about food, can all influence the likelihood of regaining weight. This is crucial information for anyone with a weight problem.

If you have a significant weight problem (and particularly if you are female) it is likely that you have come across prejudice associated with your size. There is discrimination in many areas - including employment, the media and transport. Studies show that those most likely to be prejudiced are conservative, racist men who are in favour of capital punishment and afraid of gaining weight themselves. Chapter 6 gives practical advice about how to cope with the stigma that can go with being overweight, and presents the evidence that the prejudice is unfounded.

The final chapter will help you to work out the best way to manage your own weight problem. Many people think that they are overweight, when in fact they are within the normal healthy weight limits for their height. This chapter will help you to work out whether you actually have a weight problem or not. If you do have a weight problem, then the information in this book can help you to make an individual plan. This will cover gathering information from your life, including evidence of genetics, your childhood and your present attitude to food (and whether there is an emotional/uncontrolled/restrained component to eating). The plan covers goal weight, changing what is eaten, attitudes to food, exercise/activity, social support, weight monitoring and coping with stigma. There is also advice about the food budget, meal planning, alcohol, and how to adapt favourite foods to produce healthier, less calorific meals.

Chapter 1: Global weight gain is not due to greed - why we're getting bigger

In 2010, *The Washington Post* reported that the latest threat to US national security was obesity. Thirty per cent of young adults aged 17 to 24 were too overweight to serve in the military. There are a myriad of statistics, produced by various bodies, showing that obesity is becoming a problem around the world. The actual figures vary from one study to another. One reason for this is that studies relying on people to take their own measurements, show different results to those studies where measurements are made by actual researchers. People generally claim to be taller and weigh less than they actually do, which affects the results. However, in the USA and the UK, the general consensus is that around 60% of the population are now above the desirable weight for their height.

If you have a weight problem, you are definitely not alone and it has certainly not been caused by a global outbreak of greed, or lack of willpower. It is likely that you have inherited genes that will make you more prone to put on weight than other, slimmer, members of the community. Also, changes that have occurred in food availability and lifestyle in the last few decades are contributing to your weight problem. This is not to say that you will remain big. There are most certainly things you can do to combat the problem and I hope you will find helpful information further in this book. Firstly, this chapter looks at the causes of the weight gain - because if you can identify the cause of the problem, managing it becomes easier.

It's your genes

If you have a problem with excess weight, it is likely that your family and relatives are big too. Think about families you know, or take a look at famous people with their families on Google and you will find that the build of their children, brothers, sisters and parents tends to be similar. People who are plumper tend to have plump offspring. Similarly, slim parents tend to have slim children. Although people are generally aware that there is an inherited tendency with height, with tall people tending to have tall children, there is much less awareness that weight is inherited to the same extent.

You might think that the similarity of body size within family members is because they are all eating the same food? The plumper families might have a kitchen full of pies and the refrigerators of the slimmer families are stocked with celery and yoghurt?

In fact, the scientific evidence is strong that within the population, 50-70% of the difference in weight of individuals is due to genetic influences. This comes from studies of hundreds of adopted children, where a strong relationship was found between the weight of the adopted person and their biological parents, but little relationship between the weight of the adopted person and the adoptive parents. The adoptive parents might be stick thin, but if the natural parents were large, then the child grew up large. This points towards the child's genes predisposing to large size. It is most unlikely that adoptive parents will feed themselves and their other offspring lower calorie, healthier food, whilst ensuring that the adopted child is singled out for extra puddings.

Similarly, large scale studies have shown that identical twins who grow up apart have a closely matched body weight. (The references for the medical papers supplying this data are at the end of the book, if you are interested in the details.) The twins might be brought up in different environments, with different food availability and exercise opportunities, but their body sizes tend to end up the same. This indicates that genes are influential in body size.

If you and a friend overeat by the same amount, the increase in your weights might be very different, as your genes influence what happens to the extra calories. Do you think that you could eat an extra 1,000 calories a day, 6 days a week, for a total of 84 days? Dr Claude Bouchard persuaded twelve pairs of identical male twins to do just this, in an experiment which illustrated the genetic influence on weight. In his report of the experiment, he doesn't say why he only picked male twins, but I am guessing that he might have found it more difficult to persuade female twins to agree to eat an extra 84,000 calories each. The twins lived in a dormitory on the campus of Laval University in Quebec and underwent 24 hour supervision, being only allowed 30 minutes a day of limited exercise. They spent most of their time reading, playing cards and watching television. Occasionally, they were taken as a supervised group to the cinema. Each man consumed a total of 84,000 extra calories above his normal diet in this time and they all put on weight. The amount varied from 4kg (9lbs) to 13kg(29lbs). Although there was a huge variation among the group as a whole, each twin put on an amount of weight that was very close to that of his twin. The twins also resembled each other, in that their weight gain was on similar parts of their bodies.

The man who gained the most weight (13kg/29lbs) had not dissipated any excess energy (all the extra food had been stored as body tissue) but the man who only gained 4 kg (9lbs) must have only used about 40% of the extra food to make new body tissues. This shows that genes are important in deciding how a body will metabolise extra food and that weight gain is partly related to genetic characteristics. It is certainly not a "level playing field" and if you and your neighbour overeat by equal amounts, you will probably not put on the same amount of weight.

So the evidence is strong - your genes are likely to be contributing to a weight problem if you have one. Everyone is not the same and larger people are not "just greedier" than others. This does not mean to say that you are destined to put on weight because your family are large, but it does mean you might find it easier to put on weight compared to someone whose relatives are all slimmer. Nor does it mean that you cannot lose weight. The recent rise in the numbers of us getting larger is not because our genes have changed, the rise is far too rapid. More of us are gaining weight because other factors in our food and lifestyle have changed in the last few decades. These changes mean that those of us genetically predisposed to gain weight are likely to do so. It's a combination of genes that are working hard to store calories as fat, with changes in the modern way of life, that is causing the obesity problem. Later in this chapter we will discuss some of these changes, because if you know what is causing the weight to go on, it will be easier to stop it happening.

Firstly though, you might be wondering why on earth you have inherited genes that help you to put on weight? What use is that to anyone? Well, being able to put on weight easily would have been an advantage to survival in times of food shortages. Having a "supermodel" skinny body shape in times of famine, would quickly lead to death, with those that have a supply of fat to fall back on more likely to survive. A person of 17 stone (238lbs/108kg) has enough fat stores to provide energy for about five months. It also explains why populations that have had centuries of food shortages or famines, can often quickly become very obese, if their food supply changes to a more Western type of plentiful diet. Their "survivor" genes that help them to put on weight are storing the fat for the next famine.

Which genes are causing the problem? Genetic research is at a very early stage and it is likely to be a complex answer involving multiple genes. Just a few genes have been identified so far, such as the gene that causes the hormone leptin to be produced. Leptin makes us feel full and reduces appetite. There are a very small group of people who have abnormalities of this gene. These unfortunate people produce no leptin, are always hungry, never get full and become very obese. A child of nine years of age with a mutation in the gene for leptin reached 14 stone (196lbs/90kg). Fortunately, this can be treated with injections of leptin, leading to the body size and appetite quickly returning to normal. However, the vast majority of people with an excess weight problem do not have an abnormality of this gene and larger people often have high levels of leptin. Although research into genetic control of weight is ongoing, at present not enough is known about the individual genes causing the weight gain to be of any practical use to anyone with a weight problem. We know the tendency to put on weight is inherited, but the actual genes and gene combinations responsible have not all been identified.

Although genes are of crucial importance in deciding which among us are the most likely to become obese, the marked rise in obesity during the last thirty years is far too rapid to be due to changes in genes in the population. Instead, changes have occurred in our lifestyle and surroundings, which have put those with the genes that tend to put on weight at much greater risk of becoming overweight or obese.

What has changed in the last thirty years to make those of us that are genetically programmed to put on weight, actually become fatter?

It's your food

Although you might think you eat just because you are hungry, in practice this is probably not the case. Experiments have shown that what we eat and how much we consume depends on many other factors - such as food availability, accessibility, portion size, who we are eating with and the type of place we are eating in. These things influence our eating so much that some would say that eating is more of an automatic, unconscious behaviour, rather than a matter of personal choice.

The popular idea that we are totally in control of what we eat on a conscious and intellectual level, is not actually true. In the short term, signals such as the sight or smell of food, emotion, metabolic signals to the brain (such as glucose levels) as well as free will, cause us to eat or not. You might come downstairs in the morning planning to have your usual coffee and piece of toast but the smell of frying bacon and eggs greets you, as a family member has decided to make a cooked breakfast. You are no hungrier than you were a few moments ago but do you still just have your toast, or do you decide that you might alter it to a bacon sandwich?

The smell of freshly baked bread or the sight of a chocolate éclair, combined with not having eaten recently, might well lead you to eat a snack that you would not otherwise have sought out. Stopping eating can be in response to gut distension and the release of hormones in the digestive system that are produced during a meal. These short term controls keep the level of nutrients in our blood relatively constant throughout the day. In the long term, control of our eating appears to be influenced by our genes.

The comparison has been made by Dr Jeffrey Friedman (who has done much work in this area) with breathing. It is an unconscious process but you can override it and decide to control your breathing by holding your breath, but then the unconscious drive kicks back in. Going on a "diet" might have some similarity in that you can make a huge conscious effort to restrict or control eating, but sooner or later the unconscious drive might well kick back in. You find you are eating more, without being fully aware of it.

To gain weight - eat fat and fast food

If you wanted to fatten up someone without arousing their suspicion, you would do it by covertly increasing the amount and proportion of fat in their food. Of all the main nutrients in food (fat, carbohydrate and protein) fat is the most calorie-dense and least filling. You can add a lot of fat to someone's diet without them getting full.

In fact, in the thirty years from 1970 the fat intake in Europe increased by about 30% and by nearly as much in the USA. In Britain in the 1940's every 100 calories of carbohydrate food we ate (such as bread and potatoes) was associated with eating 60 calories of fat. By the time we got to the 1990's this had risen to 90 calories of fat - the proportion of fat in our diet had gone up significantly. The total number of calories we were eating went down between 1970 and 1990, as obesity rates rose, but the proportion of fat was much greater. In the USA, as well as the fat intake increasing, the total number of calories in the food supply increased from 3,200 per person per day in 1980, to 3,900 calories by the year 2000.

Obesity rates are highest in people who take the highest proportion of their energy as fat. All this extra fat in the diet is undoubtedly contributing to excess weight problems in those who are genetically predisposed to put on weight.

Where is all this fat coming from? It's not that we are spreading pounds more butter on our bread. Many food producing companies at this time, particularly in the USA, were branding food and developing new markets, often aimed at children. The increasing use of fast food restaurants has also been implicated as one of the factors contributing to the problem. In the USA, a study over 15 years of over 3,000 adults ended in 2001. It compared the body weight of those who visited fast food restaurants infrequently (less than once a week) to frequent users (more than twice a week). The frequent visitors gained an extra 4.5kg (10lbs) in weight, compared to the infrequent visitors.

McDonalds is probably unfairly often mentioned as a fast food restaurant in this context but to me its range of foods do not seem very different from any of the other similar burger chains. Although it is popular to be disparaging about McDonalds, I found it a really useful place to have a coffee when I had small children, as they always had high chairs and it was relatively inexpensive. It did not come out well in Morgan Spurlock's documentary film *Super Size Me,* when Morgan ate entirely at McDonalds for a month and documented his deteriorating physical state. Although this was by no means a scientific study, the resulting bad publicity probably led to McDonalds adding more nutritionally balanced items to their menu.

If you find yourself having to eat fast food and have a weight problem, then studying the nutritional information, which is now being made more generally available, or looking at their website, might help. For instance, a Big Mac has nearly 500 calories, 28g of protein and 24g of fat, compared perhaps to a grilled chicken salad, which has 140 calories, 20g of protein and only 3g of fat. The problems associated with fast food probably apply to all similar fast food outlets and not just McDonalds. They are only something you need concern yourself with if you have a weight problem and you also eat frequently at fast food restaurants.

As well as the rise of fast food restaurants, with the advent of the home freezer, followed by the microwave, we have had a big change in eating habits. This has taken place over a relatively short time frame. I was a child in the 60's and 70's and I can remember the first time one of our neighbours bought a home freezer. Prior to this, the only place you could keep anything frozen at home was in the ice compartment of the standard small fridge, which might just about have room for a small packet of fish fingers. We all went and looked at this newest thing in home appliances, that was proudly displayed in our neighbour's garage. It was a large chest freezer and had been filled with multiple flavours of ice cream. Generously, we were allowed to help ourselves. I remember my mother saying later that she didn't think she would get a freezer, because we didn't eat that much ice cream.

Of course, when freezers got cheaper and more widely available, we did get one. At that time, as well as being seen as a store for ice cream, you also cooked for the freezer. You made a batch of food (such as stew or spaghetti sauce) and then froze it in small portions in plastic boxes, to defrost later in the week. Over the years this use seems to have changed. I don't know many people who cook for the freezer now. I suspect that freezers are used more for oven chips, frozen peas and ready meals such as frozen pizza.

We didn't have a microwave in the kitchen in the 1970's either, so there was no choice but to buy fresh meat/poultry/fish and vegetables and spend time in the kitchen peeling, chopping and cooking. Now you can take a pre-prepared meal out of the freezer or fridge and put it straight into the microwave or oven. With more families having both parents working, this convenience issue often means that less home cooking is eaten. This change in the way we eat has been only in the past few decades and coincides with more of us getting larger.

Although we all tend to assume we eat because we are hungry, the availability and convenience of food increases the amount we eat. The analogy has been made with advertising - we tend to claim that it does not affect our buying decisions, yet the reality is that it does, and the huge amounts spent on advertising food are a testament to this. (In 2004, Dunkin Donuts spent over $60 million on media advertising and made sales of $3,400 million.)

Hunger is only one of the factors that affect what we eat - portion size is another factor that has a big influence. Portion size has increased amazingly, particularly in the USA, where much of the research into the question of weight gain has been done. Portions started to increase in the 1970's, accelerated in the 1980's and continued to rise in the 2000's, as body weight increased. The biggest increase has been in the size of cookies (biscuits) which have increased by 700%. Portions of pasta have increased nearly 500% and steaks and bagels are around 200% bigger. Fries, hamburger and soda portions are between 2 and 5 times as big as the original size. The only exception which has been found is white sliced bread, where the portion size has remained the same. Possibly this might be because white sliced bread is not often eaten in restaurants or fast food establishments and is generally still a food which is eaten at home.

Over the same period of time the portion size has gone up in some cookbooks, such as the *Joy of Cooking* in the USA, with the recipes being the same but the number of portions reduced. Fast food companies are using larger food containers and car manufacturers have had to install larger cup holders.

Dinner plates used in restaurants have also got bigger, with an increase in size of almost 25% since 1990. People serve larger portions onto bigger plates due to the Delboeuf Illusion. This is a visual illusion that means the same portion on a larger plate will appear smaller than on a small plate, so people generally compensate for this by putting more food on a larger plate. Incidentally, colour also affects how much is served. It is the contrast in colour between the food and the plate that seems to be the key factor. For instance, more pasta in a white sauce will be served onto a white plate, than pasta in a red tomato sauce. If you want someone to eat more, give them a large plate and let them help themselves to food which is the same colour as the plate.

You might think that the portion size you are given when you get your food in a fast food outlet or restaurant does not matter too much. You are a sensible person and are quite capable of judging how much to eat. In fact, people are generally not good at working out how much to eat, and eat more food when served larger portions. Experiments with adults given various portions of macaroni cheese, found that they ate more as the portion size increased, felt they needed to eat more to feel full, and felt just as full afterwards as when given an average portion. Similarly, cinema goers eat more popcorn when it is presented in a larger packet and people eat more sweets when the packet is larger. Having food readily available in large portions tends to increase consumption in most people.

Professor David Levitsky (Cornell University, USA) carried out tests on a group of students who were given lunches of vegetable soup, rigatoni pasta with tomato sauce, bread sticks and ice cream. He found that the greater the amount served, the more was eaten of all food types. Some of the lunches were standard size, some 125% bigger and some 150% bigger. Although the students were told they could eat as much or as little as they liked, they ate more as the portion size went up. He calculated that the increased size of American food portions is enough to account for the increase in the weight of the population over the past thirty years.

Holding an "ice cream social" is not an event I have heard of. Perhaps it is an American tradition that will come to the UK, in the same way as we now have sleepovers and baby showers. Professor Brian Wansink (Cornell University) held such an event to celebrate the success of a colleague. He gave his guests random bowls of either 17oz (482g) or 34oz (964g) capacity to serve themselves ice cream, with scoops that held either 2oz (57g) or 3oz (85g). I don't know how polite it is to be monitoring how much your guests consume, but after serving themselves they were asked to fill in a brief survey and then their ice cream was weighed. He discovered that those with the larger bowl served themselves 31% more ice cream without being aware of it, and the servings increased by nearly 15% when people were given the larger scoop.

As well as being a poor judge of portion size with ice cream, we are not very good at estimating the size of our drinks either. Even bar staff, when asked to pour a shot of spirit into a tumbler, pour 26% more when pouring into a short wide glass than a tall narrow glass of the same volume.

Barbara Rolls (Pennsylvania State University) experimented with students who were given potato crisps as a snack to eat in the afternoon. The portions varied from 28g (1oz) to170g (6oZ), followed by a dinner later in the day. They were told they could eat as much as they liked of the crisps and the dinner. As the size of the packet of crisps increased, the amount of crisps eaten increased, as did the combined calorie intake of the crisps and dinner. The people given the large packet of crisps ate an additional 150 calories in total, compared to the people given the smaller packet.

Having more food available means it is more likely to be eaten. Marketing experts have found that having food available in larger portions, or containers, gives the message that it is normal to eat this amount. People eat more from half full large containers than they do from completely full medium sized containers. They have also found that when the package size of foods used in meals (such as dried spaghetti) is doubled, people eat 20% more. Part of the reason is that people think the spaghetti is cheaper if it comes out of a large packet. Similarly, "buy-one-get-one-free" offers in the supermarket not only encourage buying, they also increase the amount eaten at home, as we tend to think it is cheaper. So if you are trying to lose weight, avoiding large packets of food and "buy-one-get-one-free" offers on food that is high in fat or unhealthy, might be advantageous.

Most people think that they eat because they are hungry but experiments have shown that we are actually very flexible about the amount we eat. We tend to eat what we think is normal for the occasion and can "make room" for extra food. Imagine you are in a restaurant and have ordered a large bowl of tomato soup. Suppose as you are eating it, the waiting staff keep coming along and repeatedly add an extra ladle full of soup to the bowl. Would you eat nearly twice as much soup, or would you protest that you couldn't manage it all and ask them to desist?

Professor Wansink did some famous experiments, feeding tomato soup to groups of students. Some of the students had bowls which, unknown to them, were being slowly and imperceptibly refilled by hidden tubes joined to the base of the bowls. They ate 73% more soup than the students with normal bowls but did not think that they had eaten more and did not feel any more "full" than the students with the normal bowls. The bowls were quite large - each holding 500g (18oz) of soup. None of the participants realised they were being refilled, although some said afterwards that it seemed impossible to finish the soup or eat all of it. If hunger was the only thing to influence eating, they would not have eaten so much more.

There is an upper limit to what can be eaten though. Apart from those who binge eat, or are bulimic, most stomachs can hold around 500mls (18 fl oz) volume of food, meaning that the most that an adult can generally eat is around 500g (18oz). Adding air to food to increase its volume reduces the amount we eat and reduces hunger. This was demonstrated by Barbara Rolls in a lab, where a group of men were given a yoghurt based milkshake, followed by a meal half an hour later. The milkshake had the same amount of liquid, but air was added, so the volume ranged from 300ml (10 fl oz) to 600ml (21 fl oz). The men felt fuller after the 600ml drink, compared to the 300ml drink and ate 12% less in the subsequent meal.

Accessible food gets eaten

You might see what seems like a good offer in the supermarket, perhaps "buy 2 get 1 free" on tins of biscuits/cookies. What happens then? You stand for a moment to consider the goods, work out what the offer means and then decide to buy them. You then have to put all three tins through the till and will probably be more aware of their cost than other items. When you get home, it will take you longer to unpack these tins from the car than, say, a tin of beans that you bought at the same time. Getting them to the kitchen, you are then faced with finding somewhere to store them. Chances are they will be put on a kitchen counter, or the front of a cupboard, in a highly visible space. Every time you subsequently enter the kitchen, the biscuits will be brought to your attention.

It has been shown that promotional packs of items such as cookies/biscuits and fruit juice lead to stockpiling at home and this doubles consumption. The stockpiled items come to our attention more because they cost more to buy in large amounts, it takes longer to unpack them from the car, and if storage space is short, they tend to be put in a visible place in the kitchen. Increased awareness of a particular food increases its consumption.

If food is easy to access we will eat more of it. People eat more popcorn when it is provided ready "popped" compared to when it needs popping in a pan. In cafeterias, both normal and overweight people have been shown to eat substantially more ice-cream when the lid of the ice-cream cooler or fridge is left open, rather than closed. We drink more water if the jug is on the table, rather than further away. Experiments on students at Bournemouth University found that moving chocolate bars from an accessible part of the cafeteria, to one requiring a short walk, reduced their consumption. More desserts, fruits and snacks were eaten instead. Food that is within easy reach at a salad bar is eaten in greater amounts than the less accessible items. Removing the serving spoons and replacing them with serving tongs, reduces the amount eaten by 8-16%, as it is more difficult to serve.

If you work in an office that has been given a box of chocolates, whose desk you put it on might well have an influence on who puts on weight that week. If you really wanted someone in the office to put on weight, you would put the chocolates on their desk in a glass container. People eat more chocolates if they are in easy reach, than if they have to walk a few steps to get them. They also eat more if they are easily visible, in a transparent container. People underestimate how much they eat when the chocolates are nearby and overestimate when a few steps are needed.

Some studies have suggested that very overweight people reduce their consumption of food more than average weight people, when access is difficult. For instance, eating more nuts when shelled, as opposed to unshelled, and being more likely to use cutlery than chopsticks in Chinese restaurants. Other studies have found no difference - putting the lid on the canteen ice cream cooler cuts down the amount eaten by people of all sizes.

Who we eat with affects how much we eat

Who we are eating with also affects how much we eat, although we generally don't admit it to ourselves. If you have friends around for the evening and are supplying pizza would you consciously feel you had to eat the same amount as your friends? Professor Wansink tested pairs of students who were asked to watch television together, thinking they were taking part in a study about TV viewing. A plate of pizza slices was available for them to eat. There was only a small relationship between the number of pieces of pizza eaten and how hungry the students were. There was a much higher correlation to the number of pieces of pizza eaten by the other student. However, when later asked why they ate the amount they did, the students talked about factors such as hunger, taste and fullness. Only 2.5% said that they were influenced by the amount the other student was eating.

The more people we are eating with, the more we are likely to eat ourselves. In some studies, the amount eaten increased by 33% if one other person was present, 50% more if there were two other people at the meal and so on, until those eating with seven additional diners increased consumption by 96%. We also eat more if we are with people we know, such as family or friends. Eating out with a large group of family and friends is likely to increase consumption considerably. Probably this is because group meals take longer, are generally more pleasant and might include alcohol, which could further reduce our awareness of what we are eating. People who have eaten in groups often later complain that they have "eaten too much".

This effect of eating more when in a group tends to be stronger in men than with women and is less likely to occur when the other people in the group are strangers. Perhaps then we are more concerned with the impression we are creating and don't want to look as if we are "over-doing it". When we are on our own, adults tend to eat less as the experience is generally less pleasant. We are primarily eating to relieve hunger, before we go off and do something else. The exception is among the overweight, who tend to eat more when alone. Those with a major weight problem eat more with a similarly sized person than they would with a normal sized person. Eating is not just to relieve hunger. To some extent we probably feel we are being judged by how much we eat.

If you are a man and you take a woman out to dinner on a blind date and she tucks into a generous meal of steak and chips, followed by a large chocolate dessert, what should you make of this? Actually, the correct judgment might well be that she does not find you very attractive. Women tend to eat less if they are eating with a man, especially if they judge him to be "desirable". Both men and women eat less with a stranger of the opposite sex, than if they are the same sex. There is also a tendency to eat the same amount as a companion. Both men and women tend to eat a dessert if the person they are with has dessert, especially if the companion is male. We are probably trying to make a good impression by eating less, or matching the eating of our companion.

There are also some gender stereotypes to eating. The woman who ate the steak, chips and chocolate pudding would have been challenging these, as eating larger and more "unhealthy" meals is associated with masculinity. We judge people to be more feminine if they eat smaller "healthy" meals. I am not saying that this is right - there is no good reason why a man should not order a light green salad, whilst his female companion has a huge steak dinner - it just goes against the general social stereotyping.

If someone is staring at you, you will eat less. This was bizarrely demonstrated in a study entitled *Effects of Staring on Normal and Overweight Students* by Alan Lee (University of Missouri-Kansas) who placed a statue of a human head in the vicinity of dining students. Both the overweight and normal weight students left sooner than if the head was not present and the overweight students left significantly sooner than the normal weight students. Most people don't like being watched while they eat by someone who is not eating. They may feel that they are being judged - which leads to eating less so as not to appear greedy.

Even children vary their food consumption depending on who they are with. They will eat more biscuits/cookies if they are with their brothers and sisters than if they are on their own, or with a child they do not know, when they will also be more likely to match their consumption.

Food producers get us to eat more

Why would you eat a dessert or pudding? Because you are still hungry, is probably your initial response, but as well as who you are eating with and whether they are having dessert, the description of the food can also affect whether you eat it or not. If the waiter suggested the "special" dessert today was "tiramisu" you might consider ordering it. Would you be more likely to order it if the waiter said it was, "Italian creamy tiramisu, made with finest espresso coffee and rich dark chocolate"? Tests show that when the waiting-staff describe the dessert in glowing terms those customers who are overweight are much more likely to order it, whereas more regular sized people are less affected. It has been suggested that those with weight problems might put more emphasis on external cues such as this, and slightly less on internal ones, such as hunger.

Restaurants and fast food establishments are generally well aware that their customers are influenced by many other factors, apart from just hunger, when deciding how much to eat and to spend. Bright lighting decreases time spent in a restaurant and time spent at the restaurant strongly relates to the amount of money we will spend there. Soft lighting is used because it encourages us to linger, to have an extra course or drink and because we are less self-conscious, we eat more.

Would you rather eat "red beans and rice" or "traditional Cajun red beans with rice"? Would you choose "grilled chicken" or "tender grilled chicken"? Professor Wansink found that changing just the names of these items in a canteen increased their sales by 27%, when compared to the original plainer names. The customers described the food as tastier, more appealing and containing more calories when more descriptively named, and said they would be more likely to buy these items again.

Background music can also be used to manipulate our eating habits. The sophisticated restaurant will have soft background music to encourage customers to eat slower, stay longer and order more. The fast food outlet, that wants a high turnover of customers, may play loud irritating music. This causes eating to be quicker, or even encourages overeating, without monitoring how full we are. Even the type of music played can influence our purchasing. When French accordion music is played in the supermarket, French wine outsells German, but when German bierkeller music is played, the German wine outsells the French.

If you have ever entered a competition where you are asked to describe a food product or detail its benefits, you might have wondered why you needed to do so. Bringing the consumer's attention towards a particular product can influence the amount they eat. One study asked consumers to write a detailed description of the last time they ate soup. These people went on to eat nearly 2.5 times as much tinned soup in the following two weeks, compared to a control group that did not have to write about soup.

We are also naturally designed to eat more when there is a variety of food available, as a sort of inbuilt mechanism to get a balanced diet. Eating a lot of different foods makes it more likely that we will have enough of all the nutrients we need. We eat more in a meal if it contains a variety of foods, rather than just one type of food. If one type of food is eaten, the amount we admit to liking it decreases, but the amount we like the other foods stays the same. Tests have shown that people eat more sandwiches when offered a variety of fillings, rather than just one type of filling.

Increasing variety increases consumption and this might help explain the success of the larger supermarkets that have an interest in getting us to eat more. Do you think you might buy and eat less food if it were from local shops, such as the butcher, greengrocer and baker? As the supermarket is a relatively new phenomenon, possibly the switch from buying food in small local shops, to pushing a large cart around a huge shop with more variety, has played a part in causing the rise in obesity levels? I am not saying that supermarkets are a bad thing. On a practical level, they are a very convenient way of shopping but it is worth being aware of what you are buying and taking control of what goes into the trolley, perhaps by making a shopping list and sticking to it.

If the supermarket gets too big and offers us too much choice, however, we might just lose the will to shop up and down the endless aisles. It has been shown that there is a level at which we just don't bother to buy, because the choice becomes too difficult.

This was demonstrated when a stall was set up of Wilkin and Sons jams in a supermarket, where shoppers were asked to have a taste of the jams. When the stall had 24 varieties of jams, 60% of shoppers stopped at the stall to have a sample, but only 3% of these tasters went on to buy the jam in the store. When only 6 jams were on the stall available for tasting, 40% of shoppers stopped at the taster stall and 30% of these went on to buy the jam. This study was done by Sheena Iyengar (Professor of Business, Columbia Business School) who has been blind since childhood and has achieved remarkable research into the area of choice, and how too much choice can be a bad thing. She has demonstrated that whether purchasing gourmet jams or chocolates, or undertaking optional class essay assignments, people are more likely to make the purchase, or do the essay, when the choice is limited to an array of around 6 choices, compared to a more extensive selection of 24 to 30 choices. They then go on to be more satisfied with their purchase or to write better essays, when the original set of options was limited.

Up to a certain point, if presented with a variety of dishes, or with duplicate or multiple dishes, such as at a buffet, we tend to eat more. We are not very good at monitoring how much we eat and are often surprised at how much has been consumed.

As we go around the supermarket we do not immediately eat the food we select (this tends to be frowned upon) but how hungry we are at the moment of shopping can influence the food that we buy. Average weight people who have not eaten recently and are hungry, buy more food and buy more on impulse. The situation is not the same for overweight people, who buy more if they have eaten recently and do not buy more if they are hungry. This might be because the overweight people rely less on internal signals of hunger to regulate their eating and eat for other reasons.

Do you eat ice cream when at the seaside, popcorn at the cinema, mince pies at Christmas and chocolate eggs at Easter? Sometimes we eat not because we are hungry but because the occasion demands it.

Is eating automatic?

I hope the examples we have discussed so far will have convinced you that most of the time we do not simply eat because we are hungry, but in response to other factors, such as the type of food available, how it is served and the company we are in. Some psychologists think that eating is an automatic behaviour, and is much more to do with the environment we are in, than a response to conscious decisions. We do have automatic behaviour that can be brought under voluntary (conscious) control, such as smiling, laughing, or copying another person's mannerisms, but this control is temporary and needs a lot of effort. The brain can only process around fifty bits of information each second (equivalent to a short sentence) but the total processing capacity, including the unconscious, is around 11 million bits per second. The fact that people are often not aware of how much they have eaten, and tend to eat any food that is accessible, indicates that much of our eating behaviour is automatic and we are not consciously monitoring it. In the same way we can generally prevent ourselves laughing or smiling, we can decide not to eat food, but this control is often temporary and it needs a lot of effort.

This was shown in an interesting experiment conducted by Roy Baumeister (Case Western Reserve University USA) using students who thought they had signed up for a study on taste perception. Each student came to an individual session at a lab that smelled of fresh chocolate cookies baking. They sat at a table that had two bowls on it, one containing radishes and one full of chocolate cookies and chocolates. Some of the students were asked to taste the radishes whilst the researcher was away and the other participants were told to sample the chocolate goods. They were told only to eat from the bowl that they had been allocated. In fact, once leaving the room, the researcher covertly watched the students through a one way mirror that was mostly covered with a curtain. On returning to the room, the researcher got the students to fill in questionnaires, and then pretended that they now had a wait and whilst waiting it would be helpful if they could attempt to complete a puzzle. There was also one group of students that did not get any food to taste but went straight on to try the puzzle.

The problem they were given was unsolvable. The results showed that the group that had had no food worked on average for 21 minutes, before giving up on the puzzle. The students who ate from the chocolate cookie bowl worked for 19 minutes on average, and the group that had only been allowed to eat the radishes worked for 8 minutes. The "radish only" group said that they felt more tired than was reported by members of the other groups. It was presumed that this was due to the mental effort of not eating the tempting chocolate goods. Supporting this theory was the fact that while they were being covertly observed, several of the radish group looked longingly at the chocolates, some even picked them up and sniffed them, but none of them ate them. Having to exhibit self-control over any automatic behaviour is tiring and reduces the effectiveness with which other tasks are performed. As much of eating is automatic, this explains why the people having to resist eating the chocolate became tired and gave up on the puzzle.

People are generally unaware of automatic behaviour (such as copying others' mannerisms) and therefore also unaware that the automatic behaviour is not under their control. This leads to them wrongly thinking that their inability to stay on a diet is due to lack of willpower or greed.

The amount we eat also increases when we are distracted - for instance, watching television or reading. This supports the theory of automatic eating, because it implies that even less of our conscious self is monitoring the eating, which is carrying on regardless.

If psychologists are right, and much of our eating is automatic, it follows that we would tend to eat foods that were readily accessible, pre-portioned, need little preparation and can be eaten with the fingers. Pizzas, chips, salty snacks and fizzy drinks would fall into this description and there has been a big increase in their sales over the past 25 years. Advocates of the automatic eating theory suggest that the increase in obesity could be tackled by reducing access and visibility of food (reducing portion size, limiting access to snack foods and ready meals in schools and workplaces and reducing food advertising). They suggest that the changes made might not have to be great as people are very sensitive to small changes in their environment. Eating cannot be totally automatic, or we would literally eat everything in sight, but there is clearly a large automatic component. We do not concentrate on every mouthful, or continually monitor how full we are when we are eating.

The problem with modifying the environment would be that it would also affect the thinner members of society, or the underweight, who do not need to have their access to food reduced. Those who are underweight (recovering from an illness, for example) will do better if a large variety of tempting foods are available. They should freely avail themselves of any offers to eat out with as many close friends and family as they can muster, in dimly lit restaurants with soft music playing, taking care not to invite anyone that they consider desirable.

Does subscribing to the theory of automatic eating help you to lose weight? Well, it might if you considered reducing the visibility of high convenience food; replacing the biscuit tin with a fruit bowl, storing high fat food at the back of the fridge in a non-transparent container, using smaller bowls and plates and only buying food on offer at the supermarket to stockpile if it is healthy food. However, some researchers have been known to admit that even though they are well aware that eating with several familiar people at a restaurant that is dimly lit and has soft music might lead to over consumption, and even though this is their area of expertise, when they themselves eat out they quickly get caught up in the convivial atmosphere of the occasion. Any thought of monitoring their consumption gets forgotten and they subsequently find they have over-indulged as much as the next person.

It occurs to me as I write this in early December that I am certainly vulnerable to the hazards of automatic eating associated with stockpiling. I recently bought some pretzels and cans of cola with my shopping, thinking I should start buying more groceries for the Christmas holiday period. The pretzels were "buy 3 packets for the price of 2" and the cola was at a big discount if you bought two multi-packs of cans. I didn't have anywhere in our kitchen to store them, so put them on a shelf in the utility area. Unfortunately, they are clearly visible every time I put the washing machine on. Despite having recently researched the subject of stockpiling and having read through the paper entitled *"When are stockpiled products consumed faster? A convenience-salience framework of post purchase consumption incidence and quantity"* by Chandon and Wansink, I find that I seem to have already consumed a bag of pretzels and a couple of cans of cola and its only 13th December. Neither of these items are things that are generally available in our kitchen.

Food consumption in children is slightly different to adults, because they have less control over what they eat, as it is decided by the adults looking after them. Children will eat more fruit and vegetables, for instance, when they are readily available at home, if their parents and friends eat them and if family meals are shared. They have been found to eat less fruit and vegetables when there is poverty, in single parent families or when fast food is eaten. Boys tend to eat less fruit and vegetables than girls. The more hours of television a child watches, the less fruit and vegetables are eaten. I suspect price might be underlying some of these statistics. Fresh fruit and vegetables are relatively expensive and to provide them in quantity for a large family is a significant cost.

Is refined carbohydrate making us fat? Are any particular foods more to blame?

In recent decades, the amount of refined carbohydrate in our diet (such as processed grains, refined flour, soft drinks and sweeteners) has increased. The amount of fibre has decreased, as the problem of obesity has emerged. Turning whole grains into white flour reduces the amount of fibre by 80% and the amount of protein by almost 30%. In 1967 it was discovered that high fructose corn syrup (containing fructose and glucose) could be made from corn starch. Fructose is cheap and is the sweetest natural sugar. High fructose corn syrup is now often used as a sweetener in "light" or "natural" foods and in soft drink manufacture. Is this high fructose corn syrup contributing to the weight problem, or is its emergence at a time of rising obesity just a coincidence? A review of all the current evidence by an expert panel at the University of Maryland in 2007, concluded that high fructose corn syrup does not appear to contribute to being overweight or obesity any differently than do any other energy sources. The review was supported by an unrestricted gift from Tate and Lyle.

Which foods cause us to gain weight? Dr Dariush Mozaffarian (Harvard Medical School) monitored over 120,000 healthy Americans, who were not obese at the start of the study, from 1986 to 2006, in periods of 4 year intervals. He found that in each 4 year period the average weight gain was just over 3 lbs (1.4kg). Eating potato chips (crisps), potatoes, sugar sweetened drink, processed meat and red meat was most strongly associated with weight gain. Eating vegetables, whole grains, fruits, yoghurts and nuts was most associated with weight loss.

It's your lifestyle

If you are genetically predisposed to put on weight, as well as changes in food availability that have occurred in the last few decades, there have been quite major changes in our lifestyles that may have contributed to the increase in excess weight. Our weight can be influenced by TV, our friends, the economy, having a baby and even our nationality and where we live.

Watching TV can make you gain weight

The assumption is that we are getting less exercise due to the increasing prevalence of TV's, computers, increased car ownership and the sedentary nature of many occupations. Dr Mozaffarian's study also found that weight gain was associated with alcohol use, stopping smoking, television watching and sleeping less than six hours a night, or more than eight hours a night. A similar large study of adult Finns, over nearly six years, found that those who had gained over 5kg (11lbs) weight during this time had lower levels of education and did little physical activity in their leisure time. Men with high alcohol consumption and women who had had children, were also more likely to have gained weight.

Some consider that the modern inactive lifestyle might be contributing as much to the weight problem as our change in eating habits. However, research into this area is fraught with difficulty. Measuring how much people eat with any accuracy has been notoriously unreliable, as people often under-report by as much as 30%, which is quite understandable. If a researcher asked you to list what you ate yesterday, might you feel tempted to omit the extra chocolate bar, or late night kebab?

Estimating our activity is also difficult and tends to be done by monitoring car and television ownership. In Britain, the amount of car ownership and number of hours spent watching television both went up between 1970 and 1990, as the rates of obesity rose. In America, children who watch TV for 5 or more hours a day were found to be five times more likely to become obese, compared to those who watched TV for less than 2 hours a day.

Of course, when we are sitting watching TV we are not moving much, or using up many calories, but could TV itself be encouraging us to eat more? Studies in the USA showed that obese women were more likely to eat cookies (biscuits) when watching adverts for food or drink, than when non-food adverts were screened. In adults, eating snacks in front of the TV has been associated with increased consumption of calories from fat and increased overall calorie intake, but the same has not been found for eating meals in front of the TV.

Perhaps the distraction provided by the TV reduces awareness of what we are eating? If you have a weight problem it might be worth switching the TV off when eating snacks.

Recession and stress can cause weight gain

A 1% increase in the probability of a person becoming unemployed causes a weight gain of 0.6lbs (0.3kg), and a 50% drop in real income over a year tends to lead to a weight gain of about 5 lbs (2.3kg), according to research in the USA in 2009. Factors that make Americans statistically less likely to put on weight include possessing health insurance and receiving money from family, for instance by inheritance. It has been suggested that greater insecurity of employment and pensions has occurred as obesity has been rising. There is some speculation that we are subconsciously trying to store fat to survive food shortages, that we might anticipate as a result of unemployment.

A more recent report from America into the effect of the current recession, suggests that this trend might be changing and having less money might be reducing the numbers of people getting heavier. However, this report relied on people self-reporting their own weight and height and people are notoriously unreliable, with most people exaggerating their height and reducing their weight.

Possibly the effect of a recession could cause us to get fatter if we switch to eating cheaper, higher fat foods and cannot afford so much fresh fruit and vegetables - in addition to any subconscious desire to put on weight to compensate for possible future food shortages. Alternatively, if we try to maintain the quality of our food on less money, we might do this by eating less and eating out at restaurants less often.

Having a job that is stressful has also been implicated in causing weight gain. In the UK, a long term study of over 10,000 Whitehall Civil Servants found that those who were most stressed at work were at most risk of obesity. As the stress increased, so did the likelihood of excess weight gain. Stress was considered to be present when the worker was socially isolated and did not have any supportive colleagues or bosses, and when the worker's job was very demanding but their individual control over the job was low. This was a study of British public sector office workers in London and may or may not apply to other occupations.

Can our friends make us put on weight?

One of my first jobs was as a junior doctor at a hospital in Warwickshire. As part of this job I would talk to people as they came to the hospital for operations, including always asking them how much alcohol they drank and whether they smoked. During the six months that I worked in this relatively affluent southern area, most people either did not smoke or smoked lightly and drank in moderation. The patients were generally of average body size and the proportion of overweight patients and staff seemed fairly small. The hospital canteen served a mixture of good quality foods, which included salads.

After six months, I then went to work in a Northern hospital in a more deprived area near Newcastle-Upon-Tyne. Although my (average) weight had not changed on the journey up, I noticed quite soon that I felt relatively slim. The Northern nursing staff tended to be larger - and a significant proportion of the patients were at the larger end of the weight spectrum. Alcohol intake and smoking seemed greater among the patients and staff and there was quite a difference in culture. The hospital canteen served chips and fried food. If you asked for a sandwich you would be given a "stotty" which was a very thick wedge-shaped piece of white bread with a filling of something like chicken and stuffing (made from more bread).

The wages of the hospital staff were identical to those in the South and the living costs much cheaper in the North, so the staff would have had a greater disposable income to spend on food, but the culture was quite different. Deep fried foods and pies were more prevalent and there was much more emphasis on socialising at the weekends, when groups of staff would go into Newcastle city centre. Clubbing and drinking were part of the lifestyle. The extra calories from the alcoholic drinks alone may have been quite considerable. Although, even in the depths of winter, the women never wear coats in Newcastle when they go out in the evening, so this might use up a few more calories as their bodies try to maintain temperature. When I turned up to meet ward staff in a pub in February wearing a full length coat and gloves, I was greeted with astonishment. I don't think this culture has changed much in the intervening years - in the particularly cold winter we had in 2011, the Newcastle police actually had to issue a warning to the local population to wear coats for their own safety.

During the six months I spent in the North I think I probably gained 4 or 5 lbs (2kg) in weight. Why did this happen? Could part of the reason have been because my Northern friends were a larger size? There is some evidence that having friends of the same gender, who have a problem with excess weight, increases your chances of putting on weight by social contagion. This stems from some work by Christakis and Fowler who studied the medical records of the 15,000 residents of Framingham, USA, from 1948 onwards. Every four years the residents had a medical check-up, blood tests and were asked various questions about their relatives. They were also asked to name a close friend.

Christakis and Fowler found that behaviour such as putting on weight, smoking or happiness, can spread like a virus from one friend to another. If a resident became obese, his or her friends of the same sex were nearly 60% more likely to become obese too. If a friend of a friend became obese, the resident was 20% more likely to get obese and if the relationship was a friend of a friend of a friend (3 degrees of influence) the risk still went up 10%. This occurs even if the connecting friends in the middle of the "chain" do not put on a pound. How this link jumping occurs isn't really known but one theory is that if one lot of friends gain weight, even if you don't gain it yourself, you may become more accepting of the larger form and view a larger size as a more normal state. You could then subconsciously pass these attitudes on to other friends or family, who then feel it is acceptable to gain weight.

With extra weight, the contagion is much stronger between friends of the same sex, because we relate our body image to same sex people. If a man put on weight, his female friends were unaffected and vice versa, although if a spouse becomes obese, the chance of the other spouse becoming obese increases by nearly 40%. It also depends on the type of friendship. If Mary puts on weight and she has nominated Jane as her friend but Jane does not consider Mary to be her friend, then Jane will not be affected. However, if they see each other as a mutual friend, then Mary becoming obese will increase Jane's risk of becoming obese too.

Perhaps surprisingly, there is also a genetic influence to the amount of friends we have, with some 30% of the variation in the number of friends we have due to our DNA. Our genes influence whether we are more social, or tend towards isolation.

Of course, this does not mean that if you have a weight problem you should cut out your larger friends of the same sex. Not only would this be incredibly shallow, but those with more friends were found to be happier in the same research. Happiness is slightly more contagious than unhappiness, and those who are socially isolated are statistically less happy than those with more social connections.

Apparently Fowler's favourite "Cathy" comic strip cartoon, following the publication of these findings, showed three female friends in a restaurant discussing his research. When the waiter comes over, each woman points to another and says, "She'll have a small dry salad and a cup of water."

Having a baby can make you fat

You probably don't need me to tell you that having a baby can leave you with excess weight once the child is born. A study of 3,000 women, who were not obese or pregnant at the start of the study, was done in the USA. Over five years, the incidence of obesity for those that did not have children in that time was 4.5%, for those that had one baby it was 8.5%, and for those that had two or more births it was 12.2%. It seems the more children you have, the more likely you are to put on weight.

Where you live can affect your weight

When my children were young, we used to go to NCT (National Childbirth Trust) coffee mornings that were held in our village. At such a meeting, one of the mothers said that she was very pleased, because her husband had to spend a year working in the USA and he could take his family with him. We didn't see the family for a whole year, but when they came back they had changed, from appearing to be a normal weight, to considerably plumper. At the next coffee morning, she told us all about the great time they had had in the States and then mentioned that she thought they had all put on a bit of weight while they were there. This was greeted by replies such as "Really?" and "Do you think so?" as it was a very polite village. She said that where they were staying it had been incredibly cheap to eat out in the evenings, so instead of cooking for the family, they had eaten at the local pizza house virtually every night - where there were offers such as "buy one adult meal and another adult eats free" or "children eat free if accompanied by an adult."

Our attitudes to food and our eating habits can be partly determined by which country we are living in. The French have a hedonistic view of life and they tend to see food as a source of pleasure. They choose food in moderation that they will enjoy. Americans tend to want larger quantities of food and are less interested in its quality. They have a more puritanical view of life which they think should be based on hard work and they see food as "fuel" and often as a risk factor to health. Americans are least likely to associate eating with pleasure. In contrast, studies have shown the English attitude to food to be one of worry and fear, with episodes of comfort eating and overindulgence to relieve stress.

Obesity is more common in the States than France and research has shown that the French portions are smaller than American portions in restaurants, supermarkets and recipe books. There are many more mega-sized containers of food available in American supermarkets and we know that people serve more out of larger containers than smaller ones. There are also more "all you can eat" restaurants in America and Americans eat their food much quicker than the French. In McDonalds, the French eat for 22.2 minutes on average, compared to the Americans who eat more food in less time (14.4 minutes). Americans and French give different reasons to stop eating a meal. The French will stop eating when they start to feel full, they are no longer hungry or because they want to leave room for dessert. Americans are more likely to stop eating for reasons that are less related to the actual food; such as because they had run out of drink, the TV programme they were watching was over, or they had stopped eating because everyone else had finished and it seemed normal to stop eating too.

Countries that associate food more with pleasure, such as France, tend to be the least obese. There is a school of thought that putting the pleasure back into food, instead of emphasising the health benefits, might work for some people. This type of thinking is probably behind the popular book by Mireille Guiliano, *French Women Don't Get Fat.* She urges people to enjoy food more and eat more courses in smaller portions in order to maintain a regular weight, advocating eating three course meals.

Incidentally, though by no means a scientific study, my family did try this style of eating for a short while, though none of us particularly needed to lose weight. It was when a family member was at home following a fracture and was reading this book. It seemed like a good idea to try it, as when you are limited in what you can do for health reasons, meal times become a highlight in the day. I can report that making each evening meal into a three course affair is very time-consuming and much more expensive. I found I could only manage to do it about twice a week, as making three courses took up a major part of the day.

We did have some delicious food but if anything, I think we would have put on weight had we continued, but then we're English, not French. Having been used to just having one plate of food in the evening, I found that I had to adjust to eating much smaller portions. However, I would tend to forget and eat a reasonable starter, then a main meal that resembled the size of dinner we had previously, and was really struggling to find the room to eat the dessert. There were four of us, so as well as a lot of cooking, there was also a huge amount of washing up - 12 plates instead of 4, plus extra pans and serving dishes. It was also much more costly than just producing a one course evening meal. Later in this book will be a discussion of different types of "diet" and which will suit a particular individual, but I should say that in my opinion, the overweight person most likely to benefit from this sort of regime, might well be a wealthy French woman.

The French do spend a significant proportion of their income on food (14%) compared to the Americans who spend 4% on food for the home and an additional 3-4% eating out. It is also a little worrying that Ms Guiliano gives the impression that French women are continually monitoring what they eat and going without food at one time, in order to compensate for eating a lot on another occasion. If so, this sounds a bit like the restrained/monitored type of eating which seems to be experimentally associated with more comfort eating in times of stress, compared to those who do not restrain their eating.

Comfort eating

Which brings us to comfort eating, an idea I am sure you are familiar with - eating not primarily in response to hunger, but in order to improve negative emotions or to maintain or enhance positive emotions. What do you tend to comfort eat and in what sort of situation? Take a moment to think about this before finding out if you fit into the general stereotypes.

Most likely, what you comfort eat will depend on your nationality, age and gender. For instance, the French, older people and men, tend to be motivated by positive, pleasant emotions when they eat comfort food. Their motivation for eating is to maintain or enhance these positive emotions. As people get older, positive emotions tend to dominate their decision making more than negative ones. The type of comfort food preferred varies with age and gender. Men and the over 55s tend to prefer hearty food with a higher proportion of protein, such as steaks, soups, casseroles and stews.

In contrast, women and young people tend to eat snack food of high fat and sugar content when they comfort eat. Think of the *Friends* TV series, where a tub of ice cream is produced by the female members of the cast in response to relationship difficulties. It is thought that women are more influenced by negative emotions in their decision making processes and comfort eat to relieve these emotions. Although these emotions are alleviated, there is an associated feeling of guilt. Why do women eat the sweet snacks for comfort? Well, if women are eating in response to negative stress, these types of small, high energy snacks are more easily eaten and digested than meals. As gut activity and digestion is reduced by stress, people who eat more in response to negative emotions will find this type of food easier to digest. People who eat in response to negative emotions and pick snack food that is sweet and high in fat when stressed, are more prone to put on extra weight as a consequence.

I was not very pleased to learn that women are influenced generally more by negative emotions in their decision making process and men by positive ones, until I realised that this was not necessarily a bad thing. The recent banking crisis was caused almost exclusively by middle aged men in suits - presumably all tucking into their steaks as they spent money with reckless abandon. Maybe if there had been more women on the boards of these banks, snacking on chocolate biscuits, one of them would have pointed out the possible negative consequences of spending money that they did not have.

Research into the effect of stress on eating generally has shown that mild stress tends to increase the amount that is eaten but severe stress reduces the amount consumed. Those of us who are usually restrained and controlling of what we eat tend to eat more under stress than those who are unrestrained, who eat the same or less.

Why does stress affect what we eat? One theory is that some people are particularly sensitive to the effects of the constituents of their food on brain pathways that influence mood. They may learn to self-medicate with particular foods. Some attention has been focused on the fact that a carbohydrate rich, low protein diet allows more uptake of the amino acid called tryptophan from the diet. It is then used by the brain to make serotonin, a brain chemical, the actions of which include improving mood and reducing appetite.

Tryptophan is especially plentiful in chocolate, so chocolate could work to improve mood and is then working as a comfort food. Maybe this is why J K Rowling used chocolate as a cure for the effect of "Dementors" who suck the happiness from humans, in her *Harry Potter* books - the tryptophan helping to restore happiness. However, tryptophan is also found in other foods such as oats, dates, milk, meat, fish, eggs, poultry and peanuts, so it is not necessary to eat chocolate to keep up tryptophan levels.

There is also a gender difference between the type of food

preferred by overweight men and women. When Adam Drewnowski (University of Michigan) asked obese American men and women what their favourite foods were, men preferred meat dishes, often high in fat and protein, such as hamburgers, steaks and roasts. In contrast, women tended to prefer food high in carbohydrate and fat (such as ice cream, doughnuts and chocolate) and also bread (bread being a high carbohydrate, low fat food).

Could viruses play a part in weight gain?

Some research has suggested that a type of adenovirus might be a factor in the increased prevalence of obesity. Adenoviruses are a group of viruses that can cause illnesses such as the common cold, chest infections, sticky eyes and stomach upsets. These infections are generally mild. It has been suggested that the adenovirus AD36 might be associated with the development of obesity, after it was noticed that mice and chickens infected with the virus became obese.

Some studies have suggested that adenovirus AD36 is more common in overweight children and adults than in other people, but other studies have found no such link. In my opinion, it is unlikely to be the sole "cause" of obesity, because it is often found in normal weight people. While research in this area goes on, the practical use of this information to the individual at this present time, is small.

How many of us have a weight problem?

Excess weight is generally described as first overweight, then obese (then morbidly obese at its most extreme). In the USA, where much of the research has been done, around one third of the population is classified as obese and another third is overweight, so around 60% of the people are above the desirable weight for their height. From 1998 to 2008, the number of States reporting that 40% or more of its young adults were overweight or obese increased from one to thirty-nine States.

In Britain, between 1980 and 2002 the prevalence of obesity almost trebled, with 25% of adults becoming obese, with a particular problem in Scotland and Wales. Around the globe, a similar picture of increasing prevalence of excess weight is emerging. The extent of the excess weight problem often becomes marked when calories become freely available where they were once more limited. As economic conditions improve, it is the more wealthy sections of the community that first become susceptible to obesity. In the later stages of economic improvement the rates of obesity shift and become highest among the poor.

If you are overweight, it is not your fault

The point I am hoping to make in this chapter is that if you have an excess weight problem, you should not consider that it is your own fault and due to any character flaw or greed. It is likely that you have inherited genes which will make you more prone to put on weight than other, leaner, members of the community and changes that have occurred in food availability and lifestyle, in the last few decades, are contributing to your weight problem. This is not to say that it is inevitable that you will remain big. There are most certainly things you can do to combat the problem and further into this book, I hope you will find information that will be helpful. What I want to emphasis here, is that self-blame is not only unhelpful, it is wrong.

This is by no means just an isolated opinion that I have formed from looking at the research.

A report by the World Health Organization states:

"In contrast to the widely held perception among the public and parts of the scientific and medical communities, it is clear that obesity is not simply a result of overindulgence in highly palatable foods, or a lack of physical exercise."

(WHO Technical Report - Obesity - Preventing and Managing the Global Epidemic - Geneva 2000.)

Similarly, Professor J Friedman (Rockefeller University) has said:

"To end the stigma of obesity the scientific community must communicate more effectively a growing body of compelling evidence indicating that morbid obesity is the result of differences in biology and not a personal choice."

(Friedman, Jeffrey M. "Modern science versus the stigma of obesity." Nature medicine 10.6 (2004): 563-569.)

Chapter 2: Putting the health risks into perspective and coping with medical discrimination

Why should you be concerned about any excess weight? The main reason for being worried about weight (unless you are particularly vain) is the possible effect on health. This chapter hopes to answer the question, "What are the risks to health of being overweight?" You can then decide how much this will factor into your decision making, with regard to your own situation. You will also want to know about the risks that can be associated with losing weight, and possibly how excess weight affects children. Finally, I want to talk about how to cope with the medical profession, who do not fare well in their dealings with people who have a weight problem.

Does excess weight affect adult health?

I should, perhaps, issue a warning before you continue to read this section. It is true that there is a risk to health when there is excess weight, and this risk tends to increase the larger you are. What follows includes a series of statistics highlighting the main problems. If you are feeling particularly emotionally vulnerable at the moment, you might want to skip this section or come back to it another time. I don't want to frighten anyone. Just start at the last section of this chapter (that discusses how the medical profession treat people with weight problems) instead.

Will excess weight be likely to lead to early death?

Many of the studies looking at risk of illness or early death associated with extra weight talk about, "increased relative risk." This does not mean that you will get all these conditions if you are overweight. There might just be a slight statistical increase in risk. I suppose the bottom line that most people will want to know is, "Am I likely to die prematurely because of my weight?" There are various conflicting studies into this question and the general results seem to be that weight can significantly increase the risk of dying only at the extreme end of the weight scale (possibly some effect over a BMI of 27, and with a definite risk for a BMI of 35 or over).

If you have a BMI of less than 27, then your statistical chances of early death seem to be no different to a person of normal weight. BMI stands for Body Mass Index and there are many BMI calculators available online, if you are interested. If you enter your height and weight, they will calculate your BMI (such as http://www.nhs.uk/Tools/Pages/Healthyweightcalculator.aspx).

For instance, a woman of 30 years and height of 5 ft 4 inches would need to weigh around 11 stone 4lbs (158lbs/72kg) to reach a BMI of 27, or 14 stone 8lbs (204lbs/93kg) to have a BMI of around 35. Body Mass Index can be calculated yourself, if you are mathematically inclined, by dividing your weight in kilograms by the square of your height measured in metres.

BMI is a rough guide. It can be a little inaccurate if you are particularly muscular, such as an Olympic weightlifter, when the muscle can be confused with fat, but for most people it will give a reasonably accurate result.

A large study of female nurses in the USA over 18 years (by Dr JoAnn Manson) found that the death rate in the women with a BMI of 29 or more, was more than double that of the leanest women in middle-age. However, mortality did not increase substantially until the BMI reached 27. If you find your BMI is at or above the 27 level, it does not mean you are destined to an early death. It is just a statistical increase in the likelihood over a general population, and not a personal prediction.

A more encouraging recent large study was conducted in the

USA by Neil Mehta (University of Michigan). In a thorough investigation of over 10,000 middle-aged Americans, it was found that obesity is not a large source of attributable mortality among middle-aged adults. People with a BMI of up to 34 have no increased risk of dying, compared to normal weight people. "Attributable mortality" is the fraction of deaths that would be avoided if there was no obesity. A graph of probability of dying versus BMI is remarkably flat, until a BMI of just below 35 is reached, when it starts to rise. Having a BMI of 35 or above increases mortality by around 40% in women and 60% in men, compared to mortality in those with a normal BMI (18.5-24.9). This is the relative risk.

How does the risk from weight compare to the risk from smoking?

The fraction of deaths that would be avoided in middle-aged people if no-one had a BMI of 35 or over, is around 4% of women and 3% of men. This compares to the fraction of deaths that would be avoided if there was no smoking, which is around 36% of women and 50% of men. In other words, the risk of death is increased in those with a significant weight problem and a BMI of 35 or over, but smoking is much more likely to cause a premature death than excess weight.

What these statistics seem to indicate is that being overweight or mildly obese is not likely to increase your chances of early death. When the weight problem is fairly major and your BMI is 34 or more, then there is a statistical increased risk and more cause for concern.

The individual worrying excessively about an early death is probably a waste of time, particularly if the BMI is under 27. Even if your weight is not increasing your risk of death there are many other factors that could influence your statistical risk of dying prematurely. Having a mother who has a long life makes you statistically more likely to live longer yourself - there is a strong relationship between parental and offspring longevity, with it being particularly beneficial if your mother lives to a good age.

Having a higher socioeconomic status (being wealthy) and better educated also reduces the chances of dying at an early age.

Most of these factors are not really within much control of the individual, which probably puts some of the concerns about excess weight into perspective.

I don't want anyone to be worried too much about the risk of dying - one thing is certain, that it comes to us all in the end and real life doesn't always follow statistics. What I hope this information will do, will be to help prioritise your own concerns. Take, for example, the presenter of a popular TV motoring show. He has recently written that he is concerned about his excess weight problem (particularly around his waist) and also that he is worried about his long term smoking habit. He was disappointed when a three day trip in a submarine was cancelled, because smoking is banned on these vessels and he had hoped to use the time to break his smoking habit.

On these statistics, to preserve his longevity he should probably concentrate on stopping smoking first, as a priority over any overweight problem. His large pay packet, and inclusion in the *Chipping Norton Set* (a group of wealthy, influential individuals who live in the Chipping Norton area) will statistically put him at increased chance of living longer, as it indicates higher socioeconomic status. His mother has appeared on his TV show and I believe she is now in her late 70's. If she continues in good health, this will increase his chances of longer life. I think he went to a public fee paying school, but not to university. The failure to get a degree might reduce his statistical chances of longevity.

I hope you get my point - in the end these are only statistics and any attempts I have ever seen to predict lifespan by doctors, even in those who are clearly very ill, have frequently been extremely wide of the mark and often embarrassingly so. Perhaps you should take them all with a pinch of salt. If one was to base life choices on statistics, then you could argue that the TV presenter should enroll for a university degree, stop smoking and also devote his life to caring for his mother, to ensure her life span was as long as possible, in order to maximize his own chances of longevity.

The consensus on weight and mortality seems to be that it is more of a concern at the upper end of the excess weight spectrum and having a small amount of excess weight is statistically unlikely to lead to premature death. If your BMI is 35 or over then there is cause for concern and you might be well advised to speak to your family doctor to see if they are able to help.

Will being overweight mean I'm more likely to get ill?

Being slightly overweight probably won't kill you, but could it mean you are more likely to become ill?

Much depends on the amount of extra weight you have. For those that can be categorised as "obese" and between the ages of 30 and 50, the effect of the extra weight is to add the same risk of developing long term health problems as the effect of 20 years of ageing. In other words, if your weight is enough to put you in the obese category and you are 30 years of age, you will have the same risk of developing long term health problems as a 50 year old of normal weight. Similarly, the reduction in the "health related quality of life" is equivalent to the effect of 30 years of ageing (according to Roland Sturm, Economist at RAND research institution). This means that activities and abilities are judged to be limited by the obese person and that limitation is equivalent to that which would be experienced by 30 years of ageing.

To give you some idea of the difference between the medical definition of overweight and obese - an adult of height 5ft 4 ins will become "overweight" at around 10.5 stone (147lbs/67kg) and "obese" at a weight of around 12.5 stone (175lbs/79kg). An adult of 6ft height will be "overweight" at around 13 stone 4lbs (186lbs/84kg) and "obese" at just under 16 stone (224lbs/102kg). You can check your own weight on a chart such as that shown at the beginning of chapter 7 in this book, or by putting "healthy weight chart" into a search engine such as Google.

Which illnesses are associated with excess weight? It seems that if you are in the overweight category, the excess risk is not so high. Once you get to the obese category, then statistically you are more likely to get certain illnesses. A World Health Organization report describes the obese as having more than 3 times the normal risk of developing:

- non-insulin dependent diabetes
- gallbladder disease
- high blood lipids (fats)

- breathlessness and sleep apnoea (temporary cessation of breathing in sleep).

There is a moderate increase in risk (2 to 3 times the normal risk) of getting:

- heart disease
- osteoarthritis
- gout.

There are then a whole host of diseases for which the risk of getting them is slightly raised to 1 or 2 times the normal risk if you are obese. These include cancer, especially breast cancer in post-menopausal women, and cancer of the womb and bowel (colon). There is also a slight increase in risk of reproductive hormone abnormalities, polycystic ovary syndrome, reduced fertility, low back pain and of having problems with anaesthetics. There is also a very small risk of babies of obese women being born with congenital defects, but this is a small statistical increase and most congenital defects are not related to the size of the mother.

It's quite an alarming list of conditions, but it does not mean that someone who is classified as obese on the height/weight scale will get all these conditions. It just means that there is a statistical increase in chances of suffering from one or more of these conditions, compared to a normal weight person. I think that these statistics can appear more alarming than they actually are. For instance, if I told you that being overweight would double your chances of suffering from illness X, compared to a normal weight person, you might be concerned. But if the risk to the normal weight person of getting condition X was 1 in 10,000, then being overweight would increase your risk to 2 in 10,000. This wouldn't be a worry that would keep you awake at night would it?

I did wonder when looking at some of the research and these statistics of relative risk, whether there might be an element of scare-mongering going on. Were researchers trying to make their results more eye-catching than if they had talked about the absolute increase in risk to the individual? I think this can happen when a new medicine is being marketed too. Often reports in the press will say things like, "The new medication reduces the risk of getting condition Y by 50%." This sounds good but if the chance of an average person getting condition Y is small, then any effect of the medication will be minimal.

To put things into perspective, according to statistics produced by Dr D Thompson (Economist, Policy Analysis Inc) a moderately obese man aged 45-54 years will have twice the chance of developing high blood pressure (38% compared to 18% for a normal weight man) and his risk of type 2 diabetes is 8% (versus 3% for a normal weight man of this age). His risk of getting heart disease over his lifetime is estimated at 42% (versus 35%) and his life expectancy is likely to be one year less than a man of normal weight.

If you are at the top end of the weight spectrum, the chances of running into problems are higher and there is much more chance of getting conditions such as diabetes. Research in the USA by Prof. K Narayan (Emory University) puts the absolute risk of an American 18 year old man of developing diabetes over his lifetime, to be around 20% if he is a normal weight, rising to 30% if he is overweight, 60% if he is obese and 70% if he is morbidly obese (BMI 35+). The risk for women behaves in a similar way. Whilst individual research statistics might vary, there is certainly a clear trend for there to be a significantly increased risk of becoming diabetic as weight increases, and this risk is greater at the higher weight levels.

Why are you more likely to become ill if you have excess weight? If the body has too much fat it will also need more oxygen for the extra tissue and this will lead to changes in heart function to supply the extra oxygen, leading to high blood pressure and possibly heart disease.

When you lie down to go to sleep, the extra fat on the chest and stomach area reduces the amount of air going into the lungs, which can lead to under-ventilation and temporary cessation of breathing (sleep apnoea). This type of phenomenon is more likely when the excess weight is very significant. It can lead to feeling sleepy in the daytime, with reduced drive to breathe, and increased amounts of carbon dioxide in the blood vessels. This might eventually lead to heart or respiratory failure.

"Insulin resistance" is a term that has become more popular in recent years and it is used to describe the condition where a significant amount of excess weight is concentrated around the middle of the body (central obesity). The body cannot use insulin so effectively and levels of sugar and fat in the blood increase, leading to the development of type 2 diabetes and cardiovascular disease. Some think the cause of both insulin resistance and obesity is the same, and a sustained excess of calories leads to both obesity and insulin resistance as the body tries to protect itself from high levels of fat in the blood and tissues. There is some evidence that this particular condition is associated with a high fat diet and fructose from sweetened drinks. The relevance of this term to the individual is limited, as the treatment tends to be similar to that for excess weight in general.

Men who have an accumulation of fat around their middle are more likely to develop benign prostatic hypertrophy. This is a relatively common condition of older men where the passing of urine is partially, or occasionally wholly, obstructed by non-cancerous growth of the prostate gland. A man whose waist is 43" (109cm) or more, is statistically more likely to have to undergo the operation of prostatectomy to relieve the symptoms of urinary obstruction, according to research by Dr Edward Giovannucci (Harvard Medical School).

In women, infertility is more likely to be a problem at the higher BMI categories. It has been estimated that in the USA, 25% of ovulatory infertility (problems with the ovaries) is due to being overweight, with a BMI of 25 or more. When pregnant, the woman whose weight falls into the obese category may have a caesarean section rate of around 28%, compared to 11% for non-obese women, and whilst pregnant there is an increased risk of developing diabetes, high blood pressure or having a blood clot (thromboembolic disorder). There is also a higher chance of birth difficulties and of the baby being large for its age.

Although obesity of the mother (as opposed to just overweight) is associated with increased risk of some congenital abnormalities, such as heart abnormalities, the absolute increase in risk is likely to be very small. For instance, the risk of a pregnancy being affected by a heart defect is 0.61 per thousand births greater in obese women, than in normal weight women. There is also a small increase in stillbirths in those women who have a BMI over 40. If you're pregnant and reading this, for goodness sake do not let it worry you. These are just small statistical increases which might be significant when taken over a large population of people, but are unlikely to mean much to an individual. On the other hand, if you're having difficulty getting pregnant, then addressing a weight problem might help you to get pregnant. I have included these statistics to help make life choices, not to frighten anyone.

Having excess weight is not generally associated with more psychological problems than a normal weight person. However, once the weight problem becomes significant - such as 100% overweight - there is more chance of the individual suffering from binge eating and poor body image. Binge eating tends to occur at the higher end of the BMI scale and is characterised by rapidly eating far more than a normal person would eat, whilst feeling out of control, and it is generally done alone. It is accompanied by feelings of distress and occurs at least twice a week to be classified as binge eating. Larger people who binge eat may be more likely than others to suffer from anxiety, depression or obsessive behaviour. At this level of problem it would obviously be wise to seek professional help.

There is some evidence that in women at high BMI levels there is an increased risk of depression.

Having a weight problem can certainly be distressing if it is a significant problem. A survey by Dr Cynthia Rand (University of Florida) of those who had had surgery for obesity, asked them whether they would prefer to be a severely obese multimillionaire or a person of normal weight. All replied that they would prefer to be a normal weight.

Can losing weight cause health problems?

If your excess weight is at the obese level, then losing weight should result in improvements in non-insulin dependent diabetes, blood lipid disorders (such as high cholesterol) and will reduce high blood pressure. The risk of heart disease goes down and functioning of ovaries improves, as does sleep quality, symptoms of back pain and osteoarthritis.

There are some hazards associated with intentional weight loss but these are fairly small compared to the likely benefits when the extra weight is significant. When weight loss is rapid, particularly in pre-menopausal women, there is an increased risk of developing gallstones. These can lead to pain under the right ribs, at the front of the body. The chance of developing gallstones can be reduced by limiting weight loss to no more than 2% of the initial body weight each week, by including at least 14g (0.5oz) of protein and 10g (0.4oz) of fat in at least one meal a day and by avoiding a lengthy overnight fast.

Bone density (strength) is usually raised in obese people and when they lose weight the level can be reduced, although it may still be in the normal range for the age of the person.

The problem of "weight cycling" (where weight is repeatedly gained and lost as a result of various dieting attempts) might be in itself a health risk, but there is not really any conclusive evidence that weight cycling in otherwise healthy people is dangerous to health. There is a suggestion that weight cycling might be linked to increased risk of high blood pressure, increased lipids (fats) in the blood or gallbladder disease. It is thought that those who smoke or have pre-existing disease, such as heart conditions, might put their health more at risk by weight cycling.

Fat and fit is better than fat and unfit!

There is a continuing debate among the medical community in the USA as to whether being "fat but fit" can to some extent reduce the health risks associated with obesity. The research is conflicting; with some suggesting that being fat but fit can significantly reduce the risk of illness and death. Others suggest that weight is more important than physical activity in predicting the development of ill health. Certainly, some of the conditions associated with extra weight can in themselves be improved with an increase in physical fitness. Unfortunately, the bulk of research into this question has been done with middle class, middle-aged people and predominately with men - excluding women and the elderly. Often the studies feature people who are not really that overweight because of the obvious difficulty of getting people at the extreme end of the weight scale to exercise, so they also tend to exclude those with a BMI of over 35.

Having extra weight tends to be associated with lower levels of physical fitness, with around 12% of those who are overweight and 20% of those who are obese, having a low level of fitness.

For the individual, this debate is really fairly irrelevant as most studies show that a reasonable level of physical activity at any weight is beneficial to health. Most of the health benefits of exercise come from increasing the level of exercise from low to moderate. There is less added benefit in getting to the upper end of the fitness range. More active people tend to live longer and have less risk of developing conditions such as heart disease, stroke and colonic cancer.

Thirty minutes a day, five days a week - this is often quoted as the level of exercise necessary to maintain moderate fitness, but of course individual needs vary. In this context, exercise means activities such as brisk walking, gardening, housework, swimming or cycling.

The problem with the fit but fat theory is that if you manage to get up to a moderate level of fitness by doing your 30 minutes of cycling, you probably are not in the heaviest weight category anyway. The proportion of large but highly fit people in the USA is quite low. However, it is reasonable to assume that being moderately fit is beneficial to health, whatever your weight. Whether exercise helps with weight loss, as opposed to general health, is something that will be discussed in detail later in this book, because the answer is far from straightforward.

Dr Stephen Blair, who has researched into the effect of fitness and weight on health in the USA, has admitted that he has struggled with his weight all his life. He follows a low fat diet and runs 30 miles a week but has put on 25lbs (11kg) in the past 20 years. However, he takes comfort from the fact that he is in the top percentage of people for physical fitness for his age (then 61). "I may be short, fat and bald," he is quoted as saying, "but I'm fit."

Effect of weight on children's health

There is a myth that excess weight in children is not important and they will grow out of it. Unfortunately, this is not always true. There are effects on health where the excess weight is high enough for the child to be categorised as being at an obese level of weight. If you are at all concerned about your child's weight, ask the family doctor for a proper evaluation to check whether there is a problem or not. Health problems are at the upper end of the weight spectrum, and before you start worrying you need to check whether the child is actually obese or not. The increased risks to health can make unsettling reading if you are a parent of a larger child, so I leave it to you whether to skip this section and go on to the next. I would say that statistical increase in the risk of illness does not mean that this is bound to occur in the individual child.

The child has a problem when the weight reaches the obese range, as the proportion of obese children who go on to become obese adults is around 40-60%. The obese child is statistically more likely to become an obese adult when the amount of excess weight is high and is present at a later stage of childhood, and when one of the parents could also be categorised as obese.

One study of obese 5 to 10 year olds found that over half of them had one or more of the following risk factors for heart disease - high blood pressure, abnormal amounts of lipids (fats) in the blood, abnormality in the size or function of one of the chambers of the heart, or insulin abnormalities. The extra weight of the child is now thought to have a similar effect on the body as it would in an adult.

There is also slightly higher risk of an obese child developing a range of conditions such as type 1 diabetes, low grade systemic inflammation, abnormalities of foot structure and an increased risk of developing asthma. Obstructive sleep apnoea is more likely in obese, rather than normal weight children, and they are more likely to suffer from fatty liver disease, low back pain and osteoarthritis.

Adolescents are more likely to get a skin condition called acanthosis nigricans, where they may get coloured patches on the skin on the back of the neck, armpits and over joints - weight loss will help this condition. Menstrual difficulties and early onset of polycystic ovarian syndrome are more common in adolescent girls whose weight could be classified as obese (and can be helped by weight loss). Adolescents with excess weight are also more likely to use unhealthy weight control methods such as missing meals, abusing laxatives or vomiting.

If your child has a significant weight problem, it does not mean that they will get each and every one of these conditions, there is just a statistical higher risk. If you are worried about your child, take them to a family doctor and ask for an assessment to determine whether there is a problem or not. If there is a problem, you might then ask for advice and whether a consultation with another health professional, such as a dietician or paediatrician, would be appropriate. Which brings us to our next topic of dealing with the medical profession, which I am afraid to say are not always very helpful.

Dealing with the medical profession

Unfortunately, the medical profession tends to hold the same stereotypical beliefs about excess weight as the rest of the population. Nearly 80% of severely obese people have been reported as saying that they have always, or usually, "Been treated disrespectfully by the medical profession because of my weight."

Doctors are often unaware of the genetic and environmental causes of weight gain. They wrongly blame the patient for their condition, overestimate the amount they are eating, and think that they just need to eat less and exercise more. A survey of primary care doctors (GPs) in the USA, found that over half saw their larger patients as being awkward, unattractive, ugly and non-compliant, (according to research by Dr Gary Foster, University of Pennsylvania Medical School). Many of the doctors felt ill equipped and poorly trained to treat weight problems, and this frustration at not being able to "cure" the condition might lead them to project these feelings back towards the patient.

Some doctors believe that they are helping the patient by appearing to disapprove of their condition and so provide an extra incentive to lose weight. Research by Dr Lynne MacLean (University of Ottawa) has shown that such a negative response actually alienates the patient from seeking further help, as does the provision of equipment that is too small (such as chairs or blood pressure cuffs).

It is a long time since I worked in general practice, but I can remember such an incident when a larger lady had come to consult me about a health issue. She remarked in passing that she knew her weight wasn't helping the condition but it was, "so difficult to lose weight". Until this point, the consultation had been quite friendly and I remember feeling that my instinct was to agree with her, but I stopped myself just in time, to say something that was more "professional" about how she "really ought to try". Of course, any rapport we had was lost and looking back it was completely the wrong approach and singularly unhelpful to the patient. I think, at the time, I felt that I shouldn't be seen to be condoning the problem, but all I did was alienate her. It would have been much better to agree with her that it was really difficult to lose weight and then tried to find some practical suggestions that would help.

Unfortunately, larger patients and particularly those with a severe problem, are the most common target for derogatory humour from doctors and medical students. This is especially so in operating theatres where the patient is unconscious or in obstetric/gynaecological settings (according to research by Prof. Delese Wear, Northeastern Ohio Universities College of Medicine). Examples given were of theatre staff betting how much fat they would have to remove from larger patients in order to perform a hysterectomy, and urban legends such as oreo cookies (biscuits) being found in the folds of fat of older patients.

It is not just doctors that stigmatise the larger patient. Nearly three quarters of nurses in a British survey thought that personal choices about food and activity explained why people became obese and a third thought that obesity was due to lack of willpower.

Although women whose weight puts them in the obese category are at greater risk of getting some gynaecological cancers, they are less likely to go for screening. Professor Nancy Amy (University of California, Berkeley) did a study to find the reasons for this. She found that the women were afraid they would be treated without respect and they were embarrassed at the prospect of being weighed. They wondered whether weighing was necessary and did not want to be weighed in a public area. Nor did they like the negative attitudes of staff, or want unasked for advice on how to lose weight. They did not appreciate staff trying to blame all their symptoms on their weight, or trying to use "scare tactics," such as advice to have gastric surgery.

The same study revealed that those providing the health care reported that they often didn't have the right equipment for larger patients. The scales did not register larger weights, the gowns, chairs and scanners could be too small and examination tables were not always big enough. A fifth did not have blood pressure cuffs big enough for the larger patients.

These obese women thought that staff should be trained in treating larger people and educated about obesity. They wanted respect, advice about nutrition and wellness advice. They thought that health care and preventative measures should be the issue, not their size. They felt that they could help the situation themselves by preparing a list of questions for the appointment and by being more assertive - such as asking for an appointment with someone who was "fat-friendly" when they rang the doctor's surgery. Letting the doctor know that they don't want the conversation to be about weight but want to talk about the diagnosis and treatment instead, was also suggested.

Public health campaigns organised by medical professionals may well do more harm than good in this area, as they are often badly designed - according to a review of such campaigns conducted by Sandy Szwarc (Nurse and writer for *The Washington Post*). Particularly when directed at children, they can inappropriately label large numbers of children as overweight or fat. This can lead to eating disorders, high levels of body hatred and inappropriate weight loss attempts. These types of initiatives generally have not been shown to reduce obesity problems in the long term. It would probably be better if such initiatives targeted the whole community, rather than choosing to focus on, and so stigmatise, larger children. Certain public health officials do not seem to be taking into account the impact of any stigmatisation caused by their programmes.

Our local TV news recently reported the case of a mother who had received a letter from Walsall National Health Service (NHS) Trust. It said that her 4 year old boy had been weighed and measured at his school and at 2 stone 12lbs (40lbs/18kg) he was 3lbs (1.4kg) over his weight limit for his age. The letter also said that he was clinically obese and in danger of suffering from heart disease and cancer as an adult. His mother was understandably furious. She had not been asked for permission to have him weighed or measured at school and receiving such a letter must have been very distressing. The TV pictures of the child in question playing football showed a normal sized child who certainly did not appear obese.

Why anyone should think it right to weigh and measure children at school, particularly without consulting the parents first, is beyond me. How would the staff at the Department of Health like it if they were all lined up to be weighed and measured one morning, as they got to the office, as part of a public health initiative? Or given that weight problems often occur in middle-age, would they weigh politicians without their consent as they arrive at parliament and send the results to their constituents? Of course not - it would be publicly humiliating, particularly for the larger politicians and unlikely to result in better public health.

It seems that the better way forward is for any weighing to be done only when necessary, with the patient's express consent and in a private area. Patients should be asked if they want to know their weight. Doctors should treat the presenting problem and not embarrass the patient by talking about weight every time they attend, as it will be likely to alienate them from attending further. Instead, there could be a discussion where necessary, focussing on sound nutrition (not diet) and lifestyle. This sort of information can be aimed at the whole community and not make larger individuals feel that they are being picked out for humiliation.

A national task force in the USA looked at how family doctors should treat people who are large. It recommended that there should be sturdy armless chairs in the waiting room, wide examination tables bolted to the floor to prevent tipping, large gowns, specimen collectors with handles and large blood pressure cuffs. Extra long blood taking needles and tourniquets, larger instruments for taking cervical smears and large capacity scales in a private area were also advised.

The sort of tests a family doctor might do if you have a weight problem include a variety of blood tests, such as for glucose, thyroid function, lipids (such as cholesterol) and liver function tests. They would generally check blood pressure and if an assessment was asked for and agreed to, measure height and weight to calculate BMI.

The task force said that doctors should not worry that by encouraging self-acceptance in their larger patients it would undermine efforts to encourage weight loss. Self-acceptance does not mean that the patient will become complacent and fail to follow advice about nutrition and lifestyle. It is important to preserve self-esteem. Encouraging people to live a full and active lifestyle, regardless of their weight or success in controlling it, can help them make positive changes such as becoming more active.

Which words to use to describe excess weight is something I have struggled with throughout this book. Medically speaking, the correct term is overweight, then obese, then morbidly obese at the top end of the weight range. I have had to use some of these terms, as the research has categorised weight in this way. However, in common speech "obese" or "fat" don't seem very polite terms when you are describing a specific person. Thomas Wadden (University of Pennsylvania) did some research into which words people who are large would prefer to use to describe their weight. The terms "weight", "excess weight" or "BMI" were acceptable. Less acceptable were "unhealthy body weight" or "heaviness" and least acceptable was "fatness", "excess fat", "obesity" or "large size". Some of the size activists in the USA prefer to be called "fat", "large" or "plus sized", which does not agree with Wadden's survey. It might be that the activists have a different attitude to size than the rest of the USA population. I am not sure that exactly the same results would be found in the UK, as there may be cultural differences in preferences.

It is suggested that when broaching the subject of weight, the doctor says something that is effectively asking the patient for permission to introduce the subject such as, "Would it be all right if we talk about your weight for a moment?" They could then ask their opinion, for instance, "What are your thoughts about your weight at this time?" This is less offensive than bluntly calling someone obese or fat, which might cause upset, loss of trust and a later delay in visiting the doctor when medical care is needed for other conditions.

I hope that this sort of information might be helpful to larger people when visiting the family doctor. It is just my personal opinion, but being assertive can be difficult for the NHS patient. Firstly, you might not feel your best if you are consulting a doctor and secondly, there is the underlying fear that if you "upset" the doctor they will give you or your family poorer treatment.

The British GP family doctor service used to provide 24 hour cover and was fairly accessible, but sadly things have changed. They now do not provide any urgent care at all at weekends or evenings, and alternative out of hours care seems to be virtually non-existent. Should you actually get an appointment (and in some practices this is made very difficult) sometimes you will be told to see a nurse instead of a doctor, who will diagnose and prescribe for your condition, even though she/he has no medical degree. This would be like taking your car to the garage for a service and finding the receptionist was going to do it instead of a qualified mechanic. Whilst the individual nurse might be very intelligent, expecting them to assimilate the equivalent of a medical degree just by working in the same environment is absurd.

Under this system, where it is so difficult to see a doctor in the first place, being assertive when you finally get an appointment is difficult. Larger people should not accept being stigmatised. Should they not wish to discuss weight, they could say something inoffensive such as, "I'm not here to discuss my weight today. If you don't mind, I want to talk about my medical problem." This would be unlikely to cause any deterioration in their relationship with the doctor and clearly sets a boundary for further discussion.

Is your weight affecting your health?

This chapter will have given you some idea as to whether you have a weight problem that is likely to impact on your health. Towards the end of this book, you should have enough information to decide whether you actually need to lose weight or not, and to make an individual weight loss plan if necessary. For now, if you are thinking of losing weight, you will want to know about diet. The next chapter looks at dieting and the evidence for the effectiveness of various popular diets.

Chapter 3: Does dieting work and if so which diet is the best?

"Calorie counting" was very popular in the 1970's. Little books with lists of various foods and their calorific values were common and following a 1,000 calorie a day diet was often recommended in the press for women trying to lose weight. As a teenager, I can remember trying to stick to this limit. I was a bit stocky, although not particularly overweight and at the time I thought that this was the best way to lose weight. Of course, it was an impossible regime to follow because it was not enough calories. By the time I got to the evening meal, my remaining allowance would be about 60 calories, perhaps enough for an apple. At this point I would get disheartened and give up completely, subsequently probably eating far more than I would have done had I not been trying to diet in the first place.

In the 1980's, there was a fashion for meal replacement diet aids. These were often sold through nurses, as the distributors of these products probably felt that the implication of clinical approval enhanced the product's image. A sachet of powder was dissolved in liquid and this replaced breakfast and lunch. Then a normal dinner was eaten in the evening. At this time, I was about to be married, and I was working with a nurse who was also a distributor. After mentioning to her that I would like to lose a few pounds, I was sold a box of these expensive sachets. However, after about two days I had to give up the regime. The grey lumpy drink looked and tasted disgusting and I could not work properly. I was tired and hungry and I realized that it was a ridiculous thing to do - I definitely need food. In retrospect, thinking I needed to get thinner in order to get married was quite bizarre (but not, I suspect, uncommon). I am sure my husband would neither have noticed nor minded a few pounds either way.

The F plan diet was quite popular in the 1980's and it sounded convincing. The idea was that if you ate food with high fibre content, it would make you feel full longer and feel less hungry. Anyone who remembers this diet may also remember the havoc it caused to the digestion, as it featured heavily on wholemeal bread, beans, potatoes and pulses. A couple of days of eating that diet were quite enough for many people.

I haven't tried any "diet plans" since then. For most of the short time that I tried these diets I probably would not have been classified as clinically overweight. In common, I suspect, with many young women, dieting to lose weight was probably unwisely motivated more by fashion and by feeling fat, than by actually being clinically overweight.

Since then, numerous diets have come in and out of fashion. Boxes of pre-portioned meals are now being widely advertised and "intermittent fasting" seems to be popular at the moment.

If you have a problem with excess weight, a later chapter will contain advice about how you can find out whether you need to lose weight or not. Then you can decide the best way to address the issue. This chapter looks at the effect of dieting on the body and whether dieting works at all. It also looks at some of the popular diet regimes (such as intermittent fasting, pre-portioned meal boxes and meal replacements). This background information is valuable to anyone with a weight problem.

What does dieting do to the body?

One of the most famous experiments into the effect of food limitation on the body, was done as the Second World War was coming to an end. The government in the USA knew that they would be faced with helping starving civilians in Europe, and people from prisoner of war camps who needed re-feeding. They wanted to do some research into how to best deal with the problem, so a brochure was produced entitled - *Will you starve that they be better fed?*

Thirty-six normal weight young men, who were Conscientious Objectors, volunteered to take part in an experiment into the effects of semi-starvation, at the University of Minnesota. For the first three months, they ate a normal diet of about 3,200 calories of food each day (in nutritional terms, calorie and kilocalorie (kcal) are the same). They slept in a university dormitory, ate in the Hall cafeteria, went to lectures and were given housekeeping or administrative jobs at the university. On a normal diet, they were full of energy and took part in many events such as music or drama groups and led a full social life.

At the end of the three month period, they were switched to a diet that was around 1,800 calories each day, which was similar to that being eaten by many people in Europe at that time. This lasted for six months. They had their food in two meals at 8am and 6pm, apart from Sundays, when they had one slightly larger meal at lunch time. A typical meal could consist of a small bowl of farina (a warm wheat based cereal), two slices of toast, a dish of fried potatoes, a dish of jello (jelly), a little jam and a small glass of milk. The diet was designed to resemble that being eaten in much of Europe and to produce a weight loss at the rate of 2.5lbs (1.1kg) per week. Each week, the amount of food the individual got the subsequent week was modified, depending on how well they were doing in meeting the 2.5lb weight loss, and the variation was met with slices of bread. This caused some upset at meal times, when one man would get up to five slices of bread and another only one slice.

During their time at the University, the men were also required to walk twenty-two miles each week. They were continually monitored with medical and psychological tests by Dr Ancel Keys.

On this lower calorie regime they became irritable and did not tolerate the cold well, needing extra blankets even in the summer. Weakness was a problem and one man got stuck in a revolving door, as he did not have the strength to push it around. Another man described how they would look for driveways when they crossed the street, so that they wouldn't have to step up the kerb at the other side of the street, so poor was their energy level. Some developed symptoms such as hair loss, dizziness, ringing in the ears and reduced coordination, and some had to discontinue going to classes as they didn't have enough energy. They became obsessed with food and several started collecting cookery books - one had nearly a hundred by the time the experiment ended. Food became the most important thing in their lives, with most of them eating slowly and in a ritualised way, sometimes diluting the food with water to make it appear more. One man described how he might go to watch a film - he wouldn't pay much attention to the plot but he noticed every time the characters ate and what they ate. Another recalled how he saw a young boy cycling quickly down the road and remembered thinking, "He's probably going home for his supper." He then felt, for a moment, full of irrational hatred for the boy.

They lost interest in dating, became less sociable and noticeably gaunt (with sunken faces and protruding ribs) although they began to think that everyone else was too fat, rather than it was themselves who were too thin.

Personality testing showed that they had a significant increase in symptoms such as depression throughout this period. Most of the men had periods when they were emotionally distressed or depressed. The average weight of the men at the end of this time was around 8 stone 4lbs (116lbs/53kg) - by most measures this is underweight.

Two men were dropped from the study as they could not cope with the food restriction. One bought sundaes from a local store and then stole and ate several raw swedes (rutabagas) and ate scraps from bins. The other also ate from bins and ate a large quantity of gum. Both had short stays in a psychiatric ward at the university.

The other men managed to stick to the regime, partly because they thought that it would benefit the starving people in Europe, and partly because they had a lot of faith in Dr Ancel Keys who was monitoring their progress. It was a very difficult regime to stick to and Dr Keys is quoted as saying to his wife when he got home, "What am I doing to these young men? I had no idea it was going to be this hard."

After this period was a re-feeding period, when the men were divided into groups and given an additional calorie allowance, varying from 400 to 1600 extra calories. It quickly became obvious that this was not enough and the rate of recovery was too slow, so an extra 800 calories a day was added on top of these amounts. It was calculated that those living in Europe would need around 4,000 calories a day to recover from semi-starvation and rebuild their strength.

The study ended in October 1945 but twelve men were persuaded to stay at the lab for another eight weeks so that their monitoring could continue. They could then eat what they liked and were warned not to overindulge in food. Despite this, one man had to have his stomach pumped after he overdid the eating. Another was sick on the bus after he had eaten several meals on the first day of free eating. They were surprised how difficult the transition back to unlimited food was - on average they were then eating 5,000 calories a day and on some occasions up to 11,500 calories a day. They felt they had a sensation of hunger that could not be satisfied. One noticed that he was getting better when his sense of humour returned. Most of the men did not feel "back to normal" in the first few months and they felt that it took a year or two to feel normal again. Many ate excessively after leaving the programme and one described it as a "year long cavity" that needed to be filled. In all, full recovery took about two years but there did not seem to be any long lasting effects.

This was the first time people had become fully aware of the physical and psychological effects of food restriction. The men were of normal weight when they started the programme, so you could say that this is not the same as dieting. However, many people that go on a "diet" are also technically within the normal weight range for their height. The amount of food they were eating, at 1,800 calories a day, is more than some popular diets today. This was the first real documented study of what the effect of dieting could do to people.

Dr Ancel Keys went on to discover the link between saturated fat and heart disease and was disparaging of most diets, saying they were "for the birds, if you don't like birds" and although some were harmless, "lamb chop and pineapple, that sort of thing," some were "definitely harmful". He blamed the Northern American eating habits "for making the stomach a garbage disposal unit for a long list of harmful foods" and also blamed television for obesity. He advocated the Mediterranean diet, exercise, emotional stability, not smoking, walking and swimming to avoid heart disease. He thought jogging was dangerous in older people and spent the latter part of his life living in the Mediterranean until his death at the (not statistically significant) age of one hundred.

What happens to your metabolism if you lose weight rapidly?

In 1959, eight volunteers who had been large since childhood were admitted to hospital by Dr Jules Hirsh (Rockefeller University) and put on a liquid diet that allowed them only 600 calories a day, for four weeks. The subsequent four weeks were spent on a diet that allowed them just enough food to maintain their new weights. Dr Hirsh was studying fat cells and found that the volunteers' fat cells had shrunk back down to a normal size after the weight loss. It was noticed that many of the dieters had similar problems to the volunteers in Ancel Key's Minnesota experiment. They thought about food all the time and became anxious or depressed. He then discharged them from hospital and assumed they would now stay at their new weights.

Unfortunately, they all put the weight rapidly back on when they left hospital. Further study revealed that when obese people lose weight quickly their metabolism (the rate at which they use up calories) is reduced by up to 28%. This gives them a metabolic rate that is 24% less than those of a similar size who have never been overweight. In other words, if you weigh 14 stone and lose weight quickly by a "crash diet" to now weigh 12 stone, you may then have to eat about 25% less calories than a person who has always been 12 stone, in order to maintain the new weight.

The body uses food in metabolism just to maintain the body (resting metabolic rate), some energy from food is used in digestion (thermic effect of a meal) and some is used to provide the energy for activity and movement. Anything left over tends to be stored as fat. In adults, the resting metabolic rate declines with age and tends to be higher in those who are more active. Studies in twins have shown that there is a strong genetic and inherited component to an individual's metabolic rate.

In all, of the fifty people Dr Hirsh helped to lose weight, most put it back on. The few who did manage to keep it off seemed to make it their life's work and needed to continually monitor what they ate. From this, we can take it that losing weight rapidly if you need to lose weight, is not the best way to do it - it is likely that your metabolism will be reduced, meaning you need to eat less food to maintain your new weight.

Prisoners volunteer to massively overeat

Vermont State Prison was home to an experiment by Dr Ethan Sims in the 1960's, when he asked prisoners to volunteer to put on a lot of weight in order to see what happened to their metabolism. The prisoners were aiming to increase their body weight by 25% by eating as much as they could each day. A prison was an excellent setting for such research because it was easy to accurately record exactly what each person had eaten. The problem with volunteers in the community recording their diet is that records are notoriously inaccurate. I am not so sure whether such an experiment would be considered ethical nowadays. Dr Sims described his volunteers as "dedicated professional weight gainers" and claimed the project "had been designed to provide a constructive group activity for the young institutionalised men and has yielded dividends in education and rehabilitation."

Some of the prisoners managed to eat 10,000 calories in a day but it was noticed that there was a poor relationship between the amount eaten and the weight gain, with some needing to eat much more to put on weight. Most of the weight went on around their waists and they found it difficult to eat breakfast. They ate more towards the evening. At their heaviest, their metabolism went up from the 1,800kcal/sqM needed to maintain weight when they were a normal weight, to 2,700kcal/sqM needed to maintain the obese weight. The bodies of these men were trying to reduce the weight gain by using up the extra calories. This compares to those who have become obese naturally, and relatively slowly, who only need around 1,200kcal/sqM to maintain their weight.

Some of the men did not manage to put on the required amount of weight, even though they were eating more than those who succeeded. When the period of over-feeding was finished most of the men rapidly and spontaneously went back to their normal weight without having to diet.

This seems to indicate that the body will try and resist rapid weight loss (as in Dr Hirsh's experiment) or rapid weight gain (as in the prisoners) by altering metabolic rate, and the extent to which this occurs is very variable from one person to another. Rapid weight loss will therefore be much more difficult to sustain for some people than others. Weight is not a level playing field and re-gain of weight is not just due to lack of willpower.

Is slow gradual weight loss the best way?

The Pima Indians of Arizona are prone to obesity and tend to be the focus of much research in this area. They were followed over a period of three years to see what happens to their body's metabolism when weight changes occur naturally and relatively slowly. In contrast to those losing or gaining weight quickly, it was found that their change in metabolism was much smaller than predicted from their body size, and any change in metabolism was very variable from person to person. For instance, a weight gain of 15kg (33lbs) over the long term caused an increase in metabolism of 244cal/day, which is only 33 calories more than would be expected for the usual metabolic rate for that weight. This is the equivalent in food terms to half a grapefruit. Similarly, a large reduction in weight over the long term was not accompanied by much reduction in metabolism.

It seems that any change in the body's metabolism when weight is lost, is the most dramatic when weight is lost rapidly. If it is lost slowly, then the change is smaller. The implications for those wanting to lose weight are obvious - lose it gradually and avoid "crash" diets.

There is also a big individual variation in how people respond to rapid weight loss. Some will get large reductions in metabolism as the body compensates for lack of food and in others the change in metabolism will be quite small. This might explain why there is such an individual response among people eating a particular diet. A person's genes are important in determining how their body will metabolise food and any problem of excess weight is partly related to these characteristics. As we have previously mentioned, over-feeding of genetically identical twins results in similar weight gain for each identical twin of the pair, but between different pairs of twins the weight gain is very variable.

These sort of results show how much more difficult it is for some people to lose weight and keep it off than others. There is a bit of a genetic lottery going on as to how much your body will adjust the rate at which it is using up calories, in order to undermine your attempt to lose weight. Losing weight slowly over a long period of time, as opposed to following a "crash" or extreme diet, is preferable to minimise this effect.

Do "diets" actually work?

Problem of getting good data - it is virtually impossible to record what you normally eat

In general, there tends to be a problem with studying the effectiveness of diets. Many of the clinical trials only last a few weeks or months, after which the diet is then pronounced a success. Of course, this is of little use to the person with a weight problem who will want to maintain weight loss over many years. Often the numbers of people in the sample trying out the diet will be too small to have reliable results, and they are frequently predominantly female. Generally, there is quite a significant dropout rate from diets and if these people are excluded from the final results, it makes the diets appear much better than they might be for most people. In addition, the results are often given as "average weight loss" but the individual results might vary wildly within the group from a large loss to a large gain. It is probably better to know what proportion of those that tried the diet managed to stay on it and actually lost weight.

Many clinical trials to determine the effectiveness of weight loss programmes also rely on people to self-report what they are eating. The alternative is to have people in a controlled laboratory environment when food intake can be carefully monitored. Of course you cannot do this for long and the numbers of people involved would be quite small. Self-reporting of food intake in the normal environment might better reflect how people generally behave, but people often under-record the amount of food they eat by about 25%. As well as under-reporting, keeping a diary also tends to lead people to eat less than they would normally consume. That extra bar of chocolate might be less tempting if you had to write it down and then have it assessed by a nutritionist. Prof. John Blundell (Leeds University) who has done much work in this field, thinks accuracy is difficult because people feel judged by nutritionists on what they eat. They are no more likely to give an accurate answer than nutritionists would give if they were asked to record how many extra-marital affairs they have had, or how much money they give to charity. He suspects under reporting in the former case and over reporting in the latter.

Another problem with looking at the results of trials is that people know their progress is being followed. Dr Susan Ash (Brisbane) put a large group of overweight men on three different calorie restricted diets and at the end of twelve weeks all three groups had lost the same average weight. The trial was concluded but the men were then unexpectedly asked to attend a follow up appointment eighteen months later. Just over half attended and all the original weight had been regained. The monitoring process or lack of monitoring may influence the results.

Results of dieting tend to be the same whichever sort of diet is followed - weight loss of 5-8.5 kg (11-19lbs) in six months, followed by partial regain

Dr William Caplan and Marion Franz undertook a review of around 75 different clinical trials aimed at producing weight loss that had been continued for a year or more. The general trend was that among those that completed the trials, those that had diet alone, diet plus exercise or meal replacement found that there was an initial moderate weight loss. This loss tended to plateau after 6 months, with the average amount lost being around 5-8.5kg (11-19lbs). After that, there is partial regain of weight, which after four years reduces the loss to an average of 3-4kg (6.6-8.8lbs).

The results were pretty much the same whichever sort of "diet" was being followed, apart from where groups were only given advice about food or only advised to exercise (with no dietary input) where minimal weight loss was found. Those in the very low calorie diet group had an initial dramatic weight loss followed by substantial rapid regain of weight. Although these results are helpful, there is a tendency to pool results and talk about average weight loss with each diet, which is not much use for the individual who wants to know whether the diet will work for them.

Once the six month plateau is reached, it is difficult to get further weight loss even when efforts to stay on the programme are made, but abandoning attempts completely tends to lead to weight regain.

After a year, there was generally no difference in weight loss between any of these diets.

Could Iceland persuade you to eat cod?

Around two thirds of long term weight loss studies are funded by the weight loss industry. This is understandable given the limitations on general medical research funding, and it is encouraging that there are some efforts being made to substantiate the weight loss claims of some of the diet companies.

There is a tendency for the "diet industry" to be viewed with some suspicion and whilst I am sure there are rogue elements in any industry, I suspect that the industry has spotted a need for help that is sadly lacking elsewhere. Having funding from the diet industry into weight loss research could, however, lead to the perception that the researchers were under some pressure to present the results in a way that shows the industry products in the best possible light. Some companies are at least trying to provide evidence that their products work though, and I think that this should be encouraged. The reality of the situation is that there is a lack of any government funded full scale trials into weight loss regimes and it looks like industry funding of trials is the most practical way forward. I should perhaps say here, that I am not being funded by any commercial organisation in the preparation of this book. The opinions within it are entirely my own and based on my review of the research.

When someone is proposing a new diet or diet plan to you, it definitely seems worthwhile asking the question, "Is this person going to have anything to gain, even if only indirectly, from me using this product?"

A team from the University of Iceland did a series of trials to investigate whether eating large amounts of cod could help with weight loss. Cod is the most important fish stock economically in Iceland. Most of the fresh farmed cod from Iceland goes to the UK, particularly that which is frozen - the fresh cod going to the French. Any evidence that shows eating cod helps with weight loss might assist the Icelandic economy. You can't blame them for trying.

Over 300 men and women with BMI's over 27 were put on four different randomly assigned energy restricted diets by Icelandic researchers. Group 1 ate 3 portions of lean fish 3 times a week, group 2 ate 3 portions of fatty fish (such as salmon) 3 times a week, group 3 took fish oil capsules and group 4 took sunflower oil capsules as a control group. The results were that there was no additional weight loss in the women. However, the young men taking either fish or fish oil, lost an additional 1kg (2.2lbs) of weight, over the short 4 week trial.

Further experiments were done with over 100 people eating variable amounts of fish as part of an energy restricted diet, this time for eight weeks. This is still a very short time to assess the success of any dietary intervention. There were three groups - one had 150g (5oz) of cod 3 times a week as part of their diet, one group had to eat 150g of cod 5 times a week and one group had no seafood. The group eating the cod 5 times a week lost 1.7kg (3.75lbs) more weight than the group with no cod, over the 8 week period.

Would this be enough to convince you to eat cod 5 times a week? Personally, I would want to see more evidence. It is a very short trial and we know that any weight loss diet to be taken really seriously needs to be shown to work over the long term. Also, most people need variety in their diet and when they have less variety they tend to eat less. Would these people, when faced with the fortieth large portion of cod at the end of the experiment be beginning to lose the will to eat much at all? Would you be able to eat 40 portions of cod over 8 weeks? At current supermarket prices, the cod would cost around £9 ($15) a week for 5 portions of fresh cod, or £5.50 ($9) if frozen, so it would not be a cheap diet either.

For reference, the current national guidelines for fish consumption are at least two portions a week, one white and one oily, for the average adult. Women of childbearing age need to take advice from the doctor or midwife about the best amount of fish to eat because of concerns about levels of dioxins and methylmercury in fish. Whilst fish is generally considered to be a healthy product, my own opinion is that the evidence for it being instrumental in assisting long term weight loss is not strong.

There is a definite need for better research into the long term effectiveness of diet products and regimes. Dr Adam Tsai (University of Pennsylvania) came to a similar conclusion after reviewing the major commercial weight loss programmes that were available in the USA in 2005. He found the evidence to support the use of major commercial and self-help weight loss programmes was suboptimal and more trials are needed. Since then there have been some efforts made, for instance by Weight Watchers, Jenny Craig and Slim Fast, to support research in this area. I have outlined the results of some of these trials below when discussing these types of products.

It is encouraging that this is being done and it would be good to see more research in this area. I do not have the time or space to review all commercial diets but have mentioned these brands because there is some evidence related to their use from clinical trials. There are lots of other weight loss companies, but the sort of questions you should ask will be similar when trying to decide whether or not they can help you. I would suggest you read the rest of the book before considering joining any commercial organisation. You need to find a method of weight control that suits you personally and later chapters will help you to decide the way forward, and whether this type of commercial help will be effective for you as an individual.

What should you ask of anyone trying to sell you a diet product or plan?

In general, anyone contemplating spending money joining a weight loss group, or buying products that claim to promote weight loss, should ask a few questions of the salespeople first. You should think twice about using the product if you are not satisfied with the answers. I would suggest you ask:

- How long has the diet plan/product/group been on the market?

- In that time, how many people have followed the plan or bought the product?

- What proportion of people who start on the plan/product give up soon afterwards?

- Of those that are left, what is the proportion that have lost weight after 1 year, 2 years and 5 years and how much weight have they lost? (Most will have lost weight after 6 months - it is the longer term results you should be interested in.)

- What clinical trials has the product or plan been included in and can I see the results?

- Is the product safe? Is there any risk to my health from this product/plan?

- Can I try a small amount of the product before I buy it or just buy a small amount first to try? (Be wary of companies that do not agree to this.)

- Can I cancel my order/subscription at any time and will I get a refund?

- How much does the product/service cost? Be wary of companies wanting your credit card details to provide several months of products that you cannot cancel. Anecdotally, I am aware of one elderly lady who thought she was giving her card details for one month's supply of pre-prepared meals but was later told she had agreed to the 3 month plan. She was charged a significant amount for this and at the end of the 3 months she had lost 2lbs. She did not like the meals when they arrived and probably would not have bought them if she had been allowed to try them first, as she felt they resembled "dog food".

- Do not allow individual endorsements, by ordinary people or celebrities in advertisements, to be the sole basis of your decision on whether to pay for any sort of weight loss help. One individual's experience is not enough to make an informed decision.

Larger companies offering online services should find it relatively easy to collect information about how many people are using their services, how many continue once they have started and what, if any, is their eventual weight loss after a reasonable period of time (at least a year and preferably longer). It might also be interesting to see if there are particular characteristics of the people who do well on their product/plan. Although some people find weight loss easier than others because of their genetic inheritance, it is possible that some types of people might do preferentially well on a diet plan/product. A consented anonymous analysis of dieters by factors such as gender, age, cultural identity, place of residence, occupation or personality profile might be worth doing, to see if there are any major indicators that can predict success or failure. This would be very useful information for the consumer.

If companies are not forthcoming with basic information about how many people use their product/plan and what proportion lose weight, then I think it is reasonable to be a bit suspicious about the efficacy of their products. If more people ask for this information, then they will be more likely to make it available, unless the product/plan is generally ineffective.

What different types of diet are available and how effective are they?

In this section, I have described some of the more well known diets and I have included the evidence that I can find for their effectiveness. This is for your interest - some of them can be quite dangerous. I am certainly not suggesting that you try them all out or make any decisions about how you can manage any weight problem of your own from this list. I hope that once you have read the next few chapters about the effectiveness or not of exercise, and how people who lose weight manage to keep it off, you will then be in a much better position to consider the best way forward for yourself personally.

Some of the diets/diet plans I want to discuss include those that have different proportions of fat, carbohydrate and protein, intermittent fasting (which is the current "fashionable" diet), glycemic index diets, Weight Watchers, very low calorie diets, meal replacements, pre-prepared packaged meals (also quite fashionable), wholegrain diets, diet websites and various other ideas that have been associated with weight loss claims, such as monounsaturated fats, calcium and other minerals, green tea and fruit based diets.

Proportion of fat, carbohydrate and protein?

When looking at diets there is often emphasis on the proportion of the main nutrients (protein, carbohydrates and fats) that should make up the diet. I am sure that you are already aware that foods high in protein include foods such as eggs, meat, poultry and fish. You would similarly recognise high fat foods - those with a large proportion of butter, oil or animal fats. High carbohydrate foods would be foods such as bread, potatoes and sugar.

The rationale for testing people on diets with differing proportions of these foods seems sensible. Fat is high in calories and does not make people feel "full". Although everyone needs some fat to survive it is generally less than the modern western diet contains. Would following a low fat diet therefore be helpful? Protein is generally "filling" and a reasonable level of protein might be helpful to the person wishing to lose weight.

What evidence is there that changing the proportions of these foods actually helps in weight loss?

R J Stubbs (University of Aberdeen) tested just a handful of men with food that was covertly manipulated to be either low, medium or high fat. It was found that the men ate more calories when they were given access to a diet of freely available high fat food, compared to free access to low fat food. Testing revealed that most people cannot generally recognise when their diet is being covertly manipulated - for instance, they only identify a third of high fat foods as being high fat. They are a bit better at identifying dairy based foods as being high or low fat.

We eat more calories when high fat food is available as opposed to low fat food. If you covertly wanted your family to lose weight, you would have only low fat foods available in the kitchen, so that when they opened the fridge they were presented with fruit, vegetables, poultry, lean meat etc. Alternatively, if you wanted the family to put on weight, making sure you had an array of high fat cakes, cheese and so forth clearly visible when they opened the fridge would probably be effective. (I am not actually suggesting that you do covertly modify your family's weight. It would be more ethical to get their consent first.)

Russell De Souza (Harvard School of Public Health) put over 400 people on diets with variable proportions of protein, fat and carbohydrate. The protein content was 15% or 25% of the diet - fat content was either 20% or 40%, and the rest of the diet was made up of carbohydrate, ranging from 35% to 65%. Each participant had a total energy value to their diet which was 750kcal below their baseline consumption (750 calories less than they would normally eat). After six months, participants had lost an average of 6.3 kg (14.8lbs) and there was no difference in the weight loss results from the diets. After two years, they had regained 40% of the lost weight and again there was no difference between types of diet.

An even larger trial was conducted by Dr Frank Sacks (Harvard School of Public Health) with over 800 overweight adults (BMI 25-40) who were keen to lose weight. Each person was set a diet which was also 750 kcal below their baseline consumption and they were randomly allocated to one of four groups:

- Low fat, average protein, high carbohydrate diet.
- Low fat, high protein, medium carbohydrate diet.
- High fat, average protein, medium carbohydrate diet.
- High fat, high protein, low carbohydrate diet.

The dieters were given a lot of help over the two years that the study covered. After six months the average weight loss on each of the diets was 6 kg (13lbs) and after one year they began to regain weight. At the end of two years, 80% were still on the programme and the average weight loss was 4kg (9lbs) - a third of the people had lost at least 5% of their initial body weight. There was no difference in weight lost between the four different diets.

In common with most diets, the people on these regimes lost most of their weight over the first six months and only a quarter of the people continued to lose weight between six months and one year. After six months, people found the diets more difficult to stick to and it is thought they tended, over time, to revert to their usual type of nutrient intakes.

Hunger, satisfaction with the diet and attendance at the group sessions was similar for all the diets and weight loss was strongly associated with attendance at group sessions, regardless of the type of diet. Continued contact with the dieters reduced weight regain. This either suggests that support is helpful for dieters, or that those who are unsuccessful do not tend to attend the sessions as they presumably fear being judged as "a failure". The authors of this report suggest that any type of diet can be effective when taught with enthusiasm and persistence. The editor of the New England Journal of Medicine (where the report was published) commented that it appeared the participants found complying with the nutrient limits hard to stick to, and it was disappointing that, even with these selected volunteers who were enthusiastic, well-educated and being given so much professional help, so little weight was lost.

It seems that in theory, keeping the proportion of fat in the diet low should help reduce total calories consumed and assist weight loss. The results from these tests seem to show that proportions of nutrients consumed in actual fact did not make any difference to the amount of weight lost on a diet that was calorie restricted. It might well be that people are not easily able to stick to the nutrient limits. Certainly, without professional dietary help, aiming to stick to a diet that has a set proportion of fat, protein and carbohydrate, would be quite difficult.

Taken together, the results of these trials seem to indicate that there is not a "magic formula" for the optimum loss of weight due to varying nutrient levels in the diet, as the weight loss was the same in all the diet groups. However, keeping down the proportion of high fat food in the diet as it is highly calorific and not "filling", seems sensible if trying to lose weight. People generally eat less total calories when they choose unrestricted amounts of food from food that is low in fat, as compared to having to choose from a selection of foods that are high in fat.

Intermittent fasting - great for mice

This is quite fashionable at the moment, with the Sunday newspaper supplements suggesting intermittent fasting is a "radical new way of looking at food". Intermittent fasting often involves a "fast day" followed by a "feast day", with little or no food on the fast day and unlimited food on the feast day. All sorts of claims have been made for this diet, including that it helps with weight loss, reduces cancer formation and kidney disease, lengthens lifespan and increases the resistance of brain cells in experiments simulating diseases such as Alzheimer's dementia, Parkinson's disease and stroke.

Is fasting good for the brain?

Take, for example, the claims that fasting is in some way beneficial to the brain. Much of this research has been done on mice. Rather unpleasant experiments with mice, involving injection of toxins directly into their brains, found that they all suffered similar seizures regardless of whether they were intermittently fasted or on a normal diet. However, subsequent examination of the brains, found that in some areas, more brain cells had degenerated in the normally fed mice, than in the intermittently fed mice.

Other experiments in mice show that food restriction increases autophagy in their brain cells. Autophagy is the process by which the cells are "cleansed" as components of the cells are degraded and recycled. It is thought that disruption of this process might be the cause of diseases which lead the brain to degenerate. Mehrdad Alirezaei (Scripps Research Institute) points out that the converse might be true and increasing autophagy (by food restriction) might protect the brain cells from disease. He does, however, suggest that this idea should be treated with some caution, because studies of rat brains suggest that long term starvation actually reduces autophagy in brain cells. This could damage the cells rather than protect them. So it seems to me that any protective effect of intermittent fasting on the brain in humans, is as yet just a theory that has not been adequately tested.

Will fasting make you live longer?

The rate of ageing is largely determined by genetics and we cannot do anything about our genes. The only environmental factor that has been shown to affect the ageing process (in rats) is calorie intake. Reducing the calorie intake of rats by 50-70% of what they normally eat increases their life span and reduces age related deterioration. Any evidence that reducing food consumption increases lifespan seems to be largely rodent-related. The point has been made that tests on rodents tend to make a comparison with other laboratory rodents on a normal diet. However, it is possible that the "normal" diet for a lab rodent is actually more than it would get in the wild each day. Perhaps intermittently fasting the animal is just producing the conditions that in the wild would optimise its normal lifespan, rather than prolonging its natural lifespan.

There have been other concerns about extrapolating the results of rodent tests to humans. Some strains of mice are particularly prone to kidney disease and concerns have been expressed that intermittent fasting might be prolonging their life by helping their kidney function. Extrapolating the results of animal tests to humans is not always wise. The Giant Tortoise can live over 200 years and mostly eats grasses, leaves and woody plant stems but it might be prudent to have some human evidence before emulating its diet.

I can find no convincing evidence that intermittent fasting in humans is proven to prolong lifespan.

Will intermittent fasting help with weight loss?

Unlike mice, people on alternate day fasting do not tend to eat double the amount of food on a feed day. Dr Leonie Heilbronn (Pennington Biomedical Centre) experimented with 16 normal weight people who alternated a no food day with a feast day of unrestricted eating, for three weeks. They were told that they would have to double their food intake on the feed days to maintain their weight but it was left up to them how much they ate. After three weeks they were unable to maintain their body weight and had lost an average of 2.5% of their initial weight. They did not get used to the fast days and complained of hunger, irritability and some had constipation. It seems unlikely that they could have continued on the strict alternate day regime for any length of time.

Dr A Johnstone (Rowell Research Institute, Aberdeen) found that when adults who are a normal weight fast for 36 hours, their food intake goes up 20% on the subsequent day when they are allowed to eat freely, and they prefer high fat foods for their initial meal.

These people did not need to lose weight. The attraction of intermittent fasting is supposed to be that for some people they feel better able to limit their food intake on one day, knowing that they can eat what they like the next day (of course, water is not restricted). A few trials have been done with overweight people on intermittent fasting regimes, although generally not with large numbers of people or over a long time, so the evidence for the efficacy of intermittent fasting is limited.

For instance, Michelle Harvie (Senior Dietician, University Hospital S. Manchester) did a trial with around 100 overweight or obese middle aged women which lasted six months. Half the women ate a diet which included two consecutive fasting days each week. On these days they could only eat 540 calories as two pints of milk, four portions of vegetables, one portion of fruit, a salty low calorie drink and mineral and vitamin supplements. They could not eat freely on the other days but had to eat just enough calories to maintain their weight. The other half of the women ate a continually restricted Mediterranean diet of around 1,500 calories a day. (A Mediterranean diet bases meals on fruit, vegetables and whole grain, uses olive oil and incorporates fish at least twice a week - there is less meat and sweet food.)

After six months, there was little difference in the weight loss between the two groups, but in the intermittent group 8% experienced symptoms such as lack of energy, headaches, feeling cold and constipated, and 15% complained of hunger. None of this occurred in the Mediterranean control group. 13% of the Mediterranean group reported improved health and more energy, as opposed to 6% of the intermittent group. More of the intermittent group found it difficult to stick to their diet.

This study concluded that intermittent food restriction was no easier a diet to follow than a standard diet, weight loss was about the same, but it could be a method of dieting that might suit some people.

Michelle Harvie went on to do a further trial, the results of which seem to have been widely quoted to support intermittent fasting. The sample was of 115 women who were deemed to be at high risk of developing breast cancer. They were allocated one of three diets:

- Intermittent carbohydrate and energy restricted - two days a week the dieters ate 600kcal and less than 40g of carbohydrate, then the rest of the week they ate freely from a Mediterranean diet.
- Intermittent carbohydrate diet - two days a week they ate less than 40g of carbohydrate per day and unlimited protein and the rest of the week they ate freely from a Mediterranean diet.
- Mediterranean diet, energy restricted to 1500kcal/day seven days a week.

After three months, the weight loss in the first group averaged 5kg (11lbs), the second group was 4.8kg (10.6lbs) and the third group was 3.7kg (8.2lbs) and there was a similar reduction in body fat. In the fourth month, the intermittent fast was reduced to only one day a week and the weight loss was maintained. The intermittent low carbohydrate diet was concluded to provide a novel and alternative approach to energy restriction. Whilst these findings are interesting, I am sure that the authors would not expect these to be widely extrapolated to be useful to the whole of the obese or overweight population, without further detailed study. In particular, these findings only relate to women who were selected from those with a high risk of breast cancer (not representative of the general population) and the study only lasted four months. The amounts of weight lost do not seem radically different to that on other diets generally. (Since I wrote this paragraph, Michelle Harvie has published a book, *The Two Day Diet*, the proceeds of which go to charity. It focuses on two days a week which have high protein content in the diet and suggests a Mediterranean diet for the rest of the week.)

Another study of twenty obese people who did an alternate day fast over eight weeks was done by Krista Varady (University of Illinois). On the "fast" day they ate one 450 calorie meal at lunch time, such as a vegetarian pizza, an apple and a portion of peanuts (with as much water as they wanted, of course). On the feed days they could eat what they liked but were advised to keep the fat content down below 30% of their diet and encouraged to eat a healthy diet. Four people left the trial, so the numbers were not great and there did not appear to be a control group. At the end of the eight weeks, the weight loss averaged 5.6kg (12.3lbs), similar to that which would probably have been lost on a normal calorie restricted diet.

Other small trials of intermittent fasting seem to show similar results. Ten overweight asthma patients were put on an alternate day fasting regime for eight weeks by Dr James Johnson (Louisiana State University). On a fast day, they only had one can of meal replacement shake (around 400 calories) and on the feed days they could eat whatever they liked. One dropped out because he could not manage the fast days. The rest lost an average of 8% of their body weight and some of their asthma symptoms improved significantly, but whether the improvement in asthma was just due to the weight loss or the particular diet cannot be deduced from this study. James Johnson has anecdotal evidence from over 500 people who have followed a diet of free eating one day, alternating with eating 20-50% of their daily calorie requirement on the alternate days. He reports that there has been an improvement in a variety of medical conditions in these people, such as arthritis, fungal infections, heart arrhythmias and hot flushes (flashes). However, it would need a proper trial for these claims to be substantiated - many of these conditions might have got better naturally in any case.

This method of dieting can be appealing as there is not the continual feeling of deprivation that can accompany a standard diet. Dr Johnson also draws attention to an article published in Spain in 1957. Healthy people in an old people's home run by nuns experimented with intermittent fasting over three years. Of the 120 residents, half ate a normal diet and the other half ate 900 calories a day on even days of the month (as one litre of milk and half a kilo of fresh fruit) and on odd days they ate a diet of 2,300 calories. This averages out at 1,600 calories a day and is the same as that which would normally be consumed by a person of this age. There was not any change in weight of the intermittent fasted group and the number of deaths in this group was not statistically different from the normal eaters. However, they did spend less time sick in the infirmary, at 123 days compared to 219 days for the normal eaters. Although the improvement in health could be due to the intermittent fasting, it seems to me that it could also possibly be attributed to any health effect of all the milk and fruit.

What happens if you fast all day and, after not eating food for 20 hours, eat all your food as one evening meal?

Twenty-one normal weight people volunteered to find the answer. For one period of eight weeks they ate three meals a day and for another eight weeks they ate all their food in the evening. Six dropped out of the study and the rest found it difficult, as they were hungry and could not get used to this method of eating. There did not seem to be any health benefits and they lost a small amount (1.4kg/3lbs) of weight. This study by Kim Stote (Human Nutrition Research Centre, US Dept of Agriculture) was not designed to focus on weight loss but to see if eating all the day's food as one meal had any health benefits - it did not, and the participants had a problem with hunger.

Total starvation - extremely dangerous

Dr A Johnstone (Rowell Research Inst.) did 3 small studies - each was of 6 obese men, who completed either 6 days of consecutive total starvation, or 3 weeks of a very low calorie diet or 6 weeks on a low calorie diet. It was found that the fasting men lost weight (up to 5% loss in 6 days), became fatigued and reduced their activity levels. This also occurred, though to a lesser extent, among those on a very low calorie diet. It was not a healthy weight loss - minimal fat tissue was lost in the starving men and most of the loss was of lean protein tissue (such as muscle).

Continuous fasting can certainly be very dangerous to health and should not be attempted without medical supervision - these men had residential supervision for 34 days in total. The men did not get used to being without food and became hungrier as the fast went on. A year later, the men on the low calorie or very low calorie diet had regained all the weight that they had lost, but the men who had fasted maintained their weight loss. The researchers thought this might be because the men who had volunteered to fast might be predisposed to do well on it, or that they might be using short term fasting to control their body weight. They conclude that although fasting can lead to weight loss there is the problem of hunger, possibly negative health effects, fatigue and loss of physical activity - fasting should not be viewed as a public health weight loss strategy.

Total fasting for any length of time is very dangerous to health and should not be contemplated without continuous medical supervision as there is a definite risk of sudden death - don't even think about it! However, there is the case of an unusual man in Dundee reported in the medical press in 1973, who fasted under medical supervision for a total of 382 days with no food and only calorie free fluids. His weight went from 456lbs (over 32 stone/206kg) to 276lbs (125kg). He was initially treated in hospital where medical intervention was required to correct the mineral content of his blood, but for the rest of the time he went home and attended out-patient appointments, where his health was monitored.

Does intermittent fasting work?

As you can tell, there are a lack of good trials of intermittent fasting as a weight loss regime. In order to be sure whether this "works" for weight loss, and to check for adverse health effects, a trial would have to be done over at least a couple of years, with a control group and a reasonable number of people. There would also have to be some consensus on the amount of food eaten on the fast day and the frequency of fasting.

Any conclusion on the effectiveness of intermittent fasting for weight loss can only be speculative at this time. It may work for some people but it is possible that it could have an adverse effect on health, and it could also cause hunger, fatigue and possibly feeling cold and constipated. With the general lack of evidence I think many would be concerned to find, for instance, that the pilot of their plane was on the second consecutive day of an intermittent fast regime and might feel safer if he/she had a sandwich before take off?

I suspect that many of the people trying this method of weight loss might end up modifying it, so it ends up less rigid, and more of "I'll eat a bit less two days a week" as opposed to sticking to definite calorie limits. Perhaps some people are better able to tolerate hunger than others?

I don't think that I could contemplate intermittent fasting if I wanted to lose weight, as I need food. The nearest I have come to enforced fasting was in a medical hospital job where one of the shifts was Saturday morning to Monday evening. During the first weekend I was there, I found I was unable to access much food. Although there was a canteen, it had very short opening hours and if you were busy with patients it always seemed to be closed. Eventually, I coped by taking a large family sized packet of digestive biscuits when I was there for the weekend shifts and just eating these when starving (there were no kitchen facilities). The net effect was by the time I got home on the Monday night, I would be sleep deprived, hungry and irritable and fit for nothing until I'd had dinner and a night's sleep.

Maybe some people are more predisposed to cope with hunger and perhaps intermittent fasting might work for them? However, in light of the lack of long term research evidence, in my opinion, it is not really possible at this time to be confident of its efficacy or health effects.

G.I. – Pureed beans on shepherd's pie

The glycemic index system of choosing food to eat in the diet was devised in the 1980s. The thinking behind it was that some carbohydrate foods (those with a high glycemic index or GI value) are rapidly digested and absorbed, or quickly turned to glucose. Advocates of this diet recommend avoiding these high GI foods and instead eating low GI foods which take longer to digest.

The calculating of the GI index of different foods is horribly complicated and involves the body's response to a test amount of the food. It is derived from the graph of blood glucose plotted for two hours after the food is eaten. To avoid the followers of the GI diet having to have a lot of blood tests, tables of average GI values of various foods have been produced.

To make matters even worse, there are also figures provided for the average glycemic load of the different foods. Glycemic load is the weighted average glycemic index of individual foods multiplied by the percentage of dietary energy as carbohydrate. This is supposed to reflect the actual impact of food with different nutritional components on the glycemic response. For instance, a carrot has a high glycemic index of 71 but if you eat a 55g (2oz) portion, this works out as a glycemic load of 3.8, which is acceptable. In contrast, a baked potato has a high glycemic index of 85 and a 110g (4oz) portion has a high glycemic load of 20, making it less acceptable to glycemic followers.

By now, you are likely to have lost the will to contemplate the glycemic diet unless you are either a chemist or a mathematician but there are tables available that list the foods and their values.

Why would anyone go to the trouble of doing all these calculations? The theory is that high GI foods are rapidly digested and blood glucose concentrations rise to levels up to twice that found with low GI foods. The higher glucose levels are thought to cause increased release of the hormone insulin, which acts via metabolic routes to stimulate fat storage in the body. Between 2 and 4 hours after a high GI food meal, this insulin then causes blood glucose to fall rapidly, the person feels hungry and possibly may prefer to eat a high GI food to rectify this. This leads to a cycle of low blood sugar, followed by eating more sugary food.

In contrast, following a low GI meal the blood sugar does not fall below normal levels, there is continued absorption of nutrients from the digestive tract and there is not the subsequent hunger. It is also thought that a person's genes could influence the individual response and the lowering of blood sugar, if any, after a meal. Low GI foods tend to be high in fibre, take longer to be digested and are thought to help avoid hunger for longer than high GI food.

In practice, following a GI diet means eating food such as fruit, vegetables, peas, beans, lentils, peanuts and whole grains and avoiding potatoes and many starchy foods such as refined grain products. It generally means eating more natural foods and less processed food. Calculations of the glycemic index of the average diet show it increased by over 20% in middle aged American women in the decade following 1980, as more processed food was included in the diet. There is some suggestion that as people in America are trying to reduce fat, they might be replacing it with food marketed as "low fat" where the fat has been replaced by a lot of sugar, making it high GI value food. Some of these low fat foods might then not be as helpful in weight loss as is the impression given from their packaging.

Twelve teenage boys who were classified as obese were admitted to Boston Children's Hospital by Dr David Ludwig and were fed meals of low, medium or high glycemic index. They had regular blood tests and were monitored to see how hungry they felt and how much they ate at the subsequent meal. For instance, the high GI breakfast consisted of processed instant oatmeal with cream and dextrose sugar. The medium GI breakfast was steel cut oats (which preserves the whole grain), cream and fructose sugar. The low GI meal was a vegetable omelette with fruit.

The boys ate 53% more food following the high GI meal than the medium GI meal and 81% more than the low GI meal. This tends to support the theory that people are less hungry after low GI meals and tend to subsequently eat less (although the omelette would have had more protein, which in itself tends to combat hunger). Similarly, another experiment by Dr Peter Leathwood (Nestle Research Centre) fed volunteers shepherd's pie with either potato topping or bean puree topping. It was found that those that had eaten the bean topping were less hungry subsequently than those that had eaten the potato topping which was a higher GI value. However, Dr Susanna Holt (University of Sydney) found the total carbohydrate content of food to be more influential in subsequent "fullness" than the GI value, in other tests of various foods.

Does the GI diet work?

A review of all the human studies comparing high and low GI foods with reference to diet and weight was done in 2002 by Professor Anne Raben (Copenhagen University Hospital). Of the 31 short term GI studies she found, hunger was reduced in 15 but increased, or was no different in the other 16. In the 20 studies which lasted at least 6 months, the average weight loss was 1.5kg (3.3lbs) on the low GI diet and 1.6kg (3.5lbs) on the high GI diet. She concluded that, as yet, there is no evidence that low GI foods are better than high GI foods in long term weight control and further research is needed before obese people should generally be advised to follow a low GI diet.

Even if there was good evidence that this diet worked, it would not be very straightforward to follow. For instance, pasta, fruit, legumes (peas, beans, lentils etc) and dairy products are generally low GI but bread and breakfast cereals can be high or low GI depending on their composition. Chocolate has a low GI value, so according to the theory you should be able to tuck into as much chocolate as you like. Unfortunately, the advocates of this diet say it is an exception and the calorie content also has to be taken into account. GI values of food can also vary depending on the crop variety grown by the farmer and on the composition by the manufacturer of processed food.

Whilst some people might find the GI diet helpful, the disadvantage seems to be that it is not the easiest to follow as you would have to keep referring to tables and probably weighing your food. However, the GI emphasis on vegetables, fruit and pulses, in conjunction with moderate intake of fat and protein probably means it is at least a fairly healthy diet. It tends to emphasize eating unprocessed and wholegrain foods which are generally healthier than processed foods.

Very low calorie diets

These more extreme diets became popular in the late 1970's and in the 1980's, particularly after Oprah Winfrey announced on her show that she had lost 67lbs (30kg) in four months using a medically supervised very low calorie liquid protein diet. She pulled a wagon full of fat, representing the weight she had lost, on to the stage. Looking back at this time years later, she has been reported as saying that she had literally, "starved herself for months" and two hours after that show she started eating to celebrate. Within two days, the size 10 jeans she had been wearing that day no longer fitted. Since then, her weight has gone up and down, apparently complicated by a thyroid problem. She is now reported to have hired a personal chef who has helped her develop a healthy eating plan low in fat and calorie restricted, based on fruit, vegetables, chicken and lean meat.

Very low calorie diets (VLCDs) usually have less than 800 calories a day. They often consist of a drink which is mixed up with water and contains protein, some carbohydrate, fat, some minerals and vitamins. Sometimes the protein is added to the diet in the form of lean meat, fish or poultry, but in both cases the person usually has to drink two litres (3.5 pints) of fluid a day in addition. There have been deaths in people using VLCD's, most of these in the 1970's, when the quality of the protein in the diet was sometimes poor. Of the deaths that happened, most were due to heart problems and occurred in people who had lost around 30% of their initial weight over about 14 months.

In the USA, these types of diet are provided by a doctor who also monitors the client, generally every two weeks. The doctor would be specifically looking for those problems that can be associated with VLCD's such as gallstones, feeling cold, mild hair loss, headaches, fatigue, dizziness, muscle cramps and constipation. In Europe, these types of diets can be bought over the counter, which makes them much cheaper, but the client is generally advised to consult their doctor before trying the diet.

Do VLCDs work?

Thomas Wadden (University of Pennsylvania and consultant for Novaris Nutrition) reviewed the studies that compared these VLCDs with conventional diets, in 2006. He found that in the short term, that is the first three months of the diet, those on VLCDs lost 16% of their initial body weight, compared to 10% in those on a low calorie diet (800-1800 calories/day). However, over two years, the weight loss was statistically the same on both diets.

Given the possible medical issues that can occur with VLCDs it seems to me that anyone would be ill-advised to use one of these diets without discussing the possible risks with their doctor first and arranging some monitoring. Would I personally recommend these diets to anyone I knew? I have to say, I would not.

Atkins and Weight Watchers

Four popular diets were compared in a trial (which lasted a year) of over 300 middle-aged overweight or obese women, by Dr Chris Gardner (Stanford University). The women were randomly allocated either:

- Atkins high protein diet - lost 4.7kg (10lbs) after one year.
- Zone low carbohydrate diet - lost 1.6kg (3.5lbs) after one year.
- Ornish high carbohydrate diet - lost 2.2kg (5lbs) after one year.
- LEARN (Lifestyle, Exercise, Attitudes, Relationships and Nutrition) low fat, high carbohydrate diet - lost 2.6kg (6lbs) after one year.

At the end of the year, the weight loss in all groups was described as modest. In all four groups, the ability of the women to stick to the diet guidelines reduced over time, especially in the Atkins and Ornish groups. The graphs of weight change for all four groups suggested that a longer follow up might have further reduced the differences in weight loss between the groups.

Diets which advocate eating high levels of protein-rich food and low levels of carbohydrate in food have been popular in recent years, but there is the worry there might be adverse effects on health. In a study of women's diet in Sweden, Professor Pagona Lagiou (Harvard School of Public Health) recorded what women were eating over a 16 year period. There were over 40,000 women, between the ages of 30-49 at the start of the study. Over the duration of the study it was found that a reduction in carbohydrate by as little as 10%, or an increase in protein by 10%, was significantly associated with increased risk of heart or circulatory disease. She concluded that low carbohydrate-high protein diets eaten over a long period of time, without considering the nature of the carbohydrates or source of the proteins, are associated with increased risk of cardiovascular disease.

This study was of all women and of their natural diet, they were not "on a diet" - so whether these results would be applicable to anyone on a high protein weight loss programme is something that needs further research.

There is, though, some concern about anyone following a high protein, low carbohydrate diet in view of these findings. Also, foods such as fruit, vegetables, cereals and so forth are generally considered important to health. Limiting them might not be the best decision for dieters.

Another study comparing diets among 160 people in the Great Boston area was done by Dr Michael Dansinger. After one year the losses were again very similar and averaged:

- Atkins - 2.1kg (4.6lbs)
- Ornish - 3.3kg (7.3lbs)
- Weight Watchers - 3.0kg (6.6lbs)
- Zone diets - 3.2kg (7lbs)

There was no statistical difference in weight loss between the diets but the amount of weight lost on each diet did go up in those people who said they were sticking to the diet, whatever its type. Many people found it difficult to stick to the diets and discontinuation rates were particularly high for the Atkins and Ornish followers. The researchers thought the results might have been better if the dieters had been allowed to choose their own diet, rather than being randomly allocated a diet.

One of the few commercial diets to try and demonstrate the efficacy of its weight loss has been Weight Watchers. Over 200 people were randomly divided into either receiving free Weight Watchers membership, or getting "self help" with weight loss, in a trial by Dr Stanley Heshka, funded by Weight Watchers. The group getting free Weight Watchers were allowed to attend weekly group sessions run by people who had been through

Weight Watchers to lose weight themselves and acted as role models. They were also provided with written educational material, social support, a weekly weigh-in, a food plan, an activity plan and a behaviour modification plan.

The "self-help" group had a 20 minute consultation with a dietician and another 20 minute meeting after 12 weeks. They were given printed information on diet and exercise and websites for health promotion were brought to their attention. This group were much more left to their own devices and within the group 14 tried using weight loss medication, 6 tried herbal products, 10 enrolled in a commercial programme including Jenny Craig, 5 joined Weight Watchers themselves and 9 mentioned an alternative plan, including Atkins. Unfortunately, because these people were all doing different things, it doesn't make for a very regular control group.

At the end of two years, the Weight Watchers group had an average loss of 2.9kg/6.4lbs (varying from a gain of 21kg/46lbs to a loss of 23kg/51lbs) and the average loss for the others was 0.2kg/0.4lbs (varying from a gain of 30kg/66lbs to a loss of 26kg/57lbs). It was concluded that Weight Watchers provides modest weight loss but was better than brief counselling and self-help. The Weight Watchers who attended most of their sessions managed to maintain an average weight loss of almost 5kg at the end of two years. From which, I suppose, you can infer either that continued attendance helps promote weight loss, or that those who lose weight might be more likely to carry on going to the meetings.

There was also a huge variation in the amounts of weight lost/gained in both groups, which seems to indicate that people do not all react in the same way to a particular diet. Given the differences our genes make to our weight, this is perhaps not surprising. This type of result seems to indicate that weight management should be tailored towards the individual. The Weight Watcher who lost 23kg/51lbs might have been very pleased with the programme and for them it undoubtedly worked, but for the dieter that gained 21kg/46lbs, any benefit seems less clear.

Weight Watchers also funded another study that compared standard general practice care with a year's free membership of

Weight Watchers, in a trial conducted by Dr Susan Jebb (University of Cambridge). In both groups, only around 60% of people finished the trial. Of those left at the end of the year, the average weight loss was 5.06kg (11lbs) for Weight Watchers, compared to 2.25kg (5lbs) for standard care through the family doctor service. Of all the people who started the programme, nearly 25% of those on standard care lost 5% or more of their body weight, compared to around 45% of those who attended Weight Watchers. From this, it seems that Weight Watchers is more likely to help dieters than standard GP care, but in this case Weight Watchers was free and in "real life" you have to pay - whether or not this affected the results, is an open question.

Finding a method of weight management that suits the individual is something that we shall come back to in later chapters and seems crucial to the likelihood of success. For the moment, you need to know what is available and I want to continue looking at some other widely advertised products, and at any evidence that they might work.

Meal replacements such as Slim Fast

Meal replacements are usually manufactured as a biscuit type bar, a soup, or a shake powder that needs hydrating. They are designed to be eaten to replace a meal or a snack of normal food. Often it is suggested that the product replaces breakfast and lunch and then a normal evening meal of regular food is eaten. The attraction is that the decision of what to eat is taken away from the dieter and the food is already pre-prepared and measured out. The replacements are portable and convenient but generally the food is not fresh or cheap. The main manufacturer of such products that should be commended for funding some studies into their effectiveness is the Slim Fast group.

According to one supermarket online advertisement, the advice they give for Slim Fast products is that, "If you want to look good for that special occasion coming up, you should pick up three snacks a day (a fruit, veggies or a Slim Fast snack) and choose two Slim Fast meals, shakes or bars, in addition to having one sensible 600 calorie meal and drinking at least two litres (3.5 pints) of water a day." At the present time, in the UK, two of the meal bars and one of the snack bars would cost a total of just under £3 ($5) a day, or around £20 ($33) a week, although you might save some money by buying less regular food.

A Slim Fast chocolate crunch bar is advertised as a meal replacement of 210 calories and costs just under £5 ($8) for a pack of four bars at present. Its major constituents are soya nuggets (23%), rice crispies (12%), glucose syrup, milk chocolate (10%), bulking agent, oligofructose syrup, humectant, sweetened skimmed condensed milk, vitamins and minerals, milk chocolate chips (3%), sunflower oil, sugar, reduced fat plain chocolate powder, flavouring, emulsifier, salt and lactose.

A Slim Fast Raspberry Shake drink costs £1.55 ($2.5) and provides 220 calories. It is nearly 80% skimmed milk, the other major ingredients are water, sugar, milk proteins, vegetable oil, thickener, stabilisers, flavourings, emulsifiers, vitamins and minerals, colours, sweeteners and antioxidant.

Do meal replacements work?

Dr Judith Ashley (University of Nevada) studied 113 women over two years. She divided them into three groups:

- One group saw a dietician who just gave dietary advice. At the end of two years they had lost an average of 1.5% body weight (plus or minus 5%). They did not get any free food.
- Free Slim Fast products were given to the second group, who saw a dietician who advised on meal replacements. They lost 8.5% (plus or minus 7%) of their body weight.
- Free Slim Fast products were also given to the third group, who saw a doctor or nurse in an office who advised on meal replacements. They lost 3% (plus or minus 7%) of their body weight.

However, of the 113 women who started the study, only 39 completed all the assessments after the two years were up, so there was quite a large dropout rate.

Another study was done using Slim Fast products by Dr Herwig Ditschuneit (University of Ulm) in which 100 people who had previously failed on an energy restricted diet were divided into two groups. There was no control group and both groups used Slim Fast products.

- One group had 3 months of a low calorie diet of regular food followed by four years of replacing one meal a day and one snack with Slim Fast products. This group lost an average of 3.3% of their body weight.
- The other group had a similar low calorie diet for the first 3 months but in this initial period 2 meals were replaced with Slim Fast shakes or soups and between meal snacks of fruit, vegetables or Slim Fast snacks were given. This was then followed by the same regime as the first group for the next four years, where one meal and one snack were replaced with Slim Fast products. This group lost an average of 8.4% of their body weight.

The meal replacements were provided by Slim Fast. It is not recorded whether they were provided free to the dieters, or whether they paid the usual price. If they were free, this might have given different results compared to dieters who have to pay for the products.

Taking this problem into account, a trial was devised in Australia by Dr Manny Noakes (sponsored by Slim Fast Institute USA and Unilever). Sixty-six people took part and this time there was a matched control group, although unfortunately the trial only lasted six months. The dieters were divided into two groups:

- One group were supplied with free Slim Fast products and they used these for two of their meals and then they ate a low fat evening meal. They were also advised to eat at least 5 portions of fruit and vegetables each day. They lost on average 9kg/20lbs (9.4% of body weight).

- The other group went on a low fat/energy diet and were supplied with shopping vouchers for food equivalent to the cost of the Slim Fast products the other group were given. This group lost 9.2kg/20.3lbs (9.3% of body weight).

In other words, the weight loss was the same whether using regular food or Slim Fast products and it was concluded that meal replacement is equally effective for losing weight as a conventional structured weight loss diet. Once the trial ended, 12% of the Slim Fast group said that they would continue to use these products. The group using the products had higher dietary calcium and this was attributed to drinking all the milk based shakes. The other group had higher fibre than the meal replacement group - their diet had included a bran cereal. It was pointed out that the Slim Fast products were convenient to use and made dining out easier in the evening.

When testing the effectiveness of these products, there is the question of whether they should be compared to conventional dieting, as in this trial, or to no dieting at all? Monitoring over 150 overweight people who were given free meal replacements for 5 years in Wisconsin, by Dr Dana Rothacker, found the men lost an average of 5.8kg(13lbs) and the women 4.2kg(9lbs). This compared to matched controls (that is similar people who were not dieting) who, on average, gained around 6.5kg(14lbs) in weight.

An analysis was done pooling the results of six studies into meal replacements by Dr Steven Heymsfield, in conjunction with colleagues, some of whom were employed by Unilever and Slim Fast. They found that by putting all the results together, the meal replacement dieters tend to lose 7-8% of their body weight. For those completing the diet after one year, the weight loss was, on average, just less than 7kg(15lbs). The comparison groups on reduced calorie diet lost 3-7% of their body weight and after one year, the average loss was just over 4 kg (9lbs).

Although these studies are interesting, there is probably a need for more controlled trials with greater numbers of people over a period of several years. This would give more information on the effectiveness of the products, whether having them free makes a difference to weight loss and would quantify the optimal length of time (if any) for which they should be used. For the moment, you will have to make your own judgement on the available evidence. These products are certainly convenient, portable and mean less decision making with regard to eating, which might reduce the tendency to eat automatically. The disadvantage is that the food is not fresh, can be costly and the variety is more limited than fresh food. There is also the problem of how to fit this food in with your lifestyle - if you are a parent, how you eat is a strong role model for your children. If at lunch time you are sitting down to a replacement shake, instead of the fresh food you have provided for the children, you have to wonder what sort of message they will take away from this behaviour. There is also the question of how easy it is to go from using these products back to regular food once the weight has been lost.

Does paying people to lose weight or giving them free food help?

Dr Rena Wing (Brown Medical School) wanted to investigate the effect of supplying free food to people trying to lose weight, and also to see if paying them for losing weight would aid their efforts. The dieters were on a standard diet regime but some were also getting some of their food for free. Others received payments of up to $25 a week for losing weight and maintaining the loss. There was also a control group that received no help.

After 18 months the group with the free food had lost 6.4kg (14lbs) on average, compared to 4.1kg (9lbs) in the groups without free food. Free food seemed to enhance weight loss in this time period. Paying people to lose weight produced no additional weight loss. The free food and payments lasted 18 months. However, after 30 months, the control group had put on 0.6kg (1.3lbs). The other groups had maintained some of their weight loss but there was no real difference between any of the groups.

Pre-packaged meals - Jenny Craig

Jenny Craig is a widely known brand that sells pre-portioned, pre-prepared food to people wishing to lose weight. The appeal of this type of diet seems to be that it is convenient, the portion control is done for you and it removes the decision making about what or how much to eat. The cost of these types of services can be quite significant. At the time of writing, Jenny Craig is advising that in the UK, it costs less than £9 ($15) a day, based on their £249 ($400) a month best value four month plan. This is a total of around £1,000 ($1660) for the four months - although, of course, your regular food bills would be less. The website does not indicate that it is possible to try the products out in small quantity first before committing to a purchase. The plan includes delivered food, weekly calls from a personal consultant, an activity plan and information about menu plans, weight loss graphs, measuring cup and shopping and eating out guides.

There have been a couple of trials done of the effectiveness of the Jenny Craig programme. In 2007, Dr Cheryl Rock (University of California) published the results of a study that divided 70 women into 2 groups.

- The first group received the whole Jenny Craig programme for free. This included the pre-packaged food, weekly one-to-one contacts with a "consultant" which was followed up with emails and 'phone calls and access to the website. They were encouraged to exercise and the programme also addressed issues such as self-acceptance, behaviour, body image and thinking patterns. They got the free food weekly, which formed the core of their meals but the women had to add their own fruit and vegetables. When they were half way to their goal weight, they reduced the Jenny Craig products to five days a week. When they reached their goal weight they were switched to a meal plan of regular food, but they could have one Jenny Craig meal a day in the transition period.

- The other group had two consultations with a dietician, 16 weeks apart. They were given printed material about diet and exercise. The dietician calculated the energy intake they would need to lose weight and gave them sample meal plans.

After a year, the Jenny Craig clients had lost, on average, 8% of their weight, compared to 1% in the other group. One participant developed gallstones but there was no evidence that this was associated with the study participation.

This seems like a good result for Jenny Craig but it is worth pointing out that the clients were getting free food and this is known to increase weight loss in itself. They were also getting more help than the other people, who just saw the dietician twice, so it depends how you view the comparison. Also there were not very many people in this trial.

Another trial with larger numbers and over two years was also done by Dr Rock in 2010, this time with over 400 women divided into three groups;

1. Jenny Craig free foods and centre based one-to-one counselling. (Lost around 8% body weight).
2. Jenny Craig free foods and telephone counselling. (Lost around 7% of body weight).
3. Two sessions with a dietician and monthly contacts (no free food). (Lost around 2% of body weight).

It seems clear that those using Jenny Craig lost more weight than those who just saw the dietician. However, those on Jenny Craig were getting the food for free and some of their success might have been due to the economic benefits to those people - and the trial picked out highly motivated individuals.

For anyone considering using these products, it would be useful to have the results of a similar trial where the participants were paying for the help, as that would more closely replicate real life conditions. It would also be helpful if Jenny Craig and similar organisations published on their website figures for the proportion that lose weight on the diet and how much they lose. With most of the orders by phone or online and with telephone counselling, hopefully it should not be too difficult to find this information. There are other commercial companies who are selling pre-prepared meals but I cannot find any evidence of medical trials of their products. It would be good if they could emulate Jenny Craig and start to do some clinical trials to demonstrate their product effectiveness.

Might eating more wholegrain and legumes (peas, beans, lentils etc) help with weight loss?

Professor Peter Williams (University of Wollongong) undertook a comprehensive review of cereal grains and legumes with respect to weight management. He found that there were not enough good studies that specifically look at the effect of higher intake of cereals or legumes on weight reduction, or that compare the effects of refined and whole grains.

He did find that:

- People who tend to eat food higher in wholegrain are less likely to be overweight.

- A lower waist circumference is associated with higher intake of whole grain cereals and legumes.

- Weight loss at a significant level can be achieved on a calorie controlled diet that is high in cereals and legumes.

Of course, some of this data could mean that people who are of normal weight preferentially eat diets high in wholegrain and legumes, rather than these products specifically assist in weight loss - more in-depth studies would be needed. What is fairly clear is that these foods are generally more nutritious and filling than their refined counterparts. Cereal grains are a good source of carbohydrate, protein and fibre and if the grain is refined, much of the fibre and nutrients are lost. Less than 10% of the USA population eats the recommended amount of wholegrain food.

So while there is not much direct evidence that eating more wholegrain and legumes will actually make you lose weight, unless it is part of a calorie controlled diet, most of it has low glycemic index. It is the type of food that might well make you feel full for longer, which is also advantageous in weight control. In the West, the most common forms of wholegrain food are oatmeal, dark bread, wholegrain breakfast cereals and brown rice. The legumes we eat most of are foods such as peas, beans and lentils.

Prof. William's work was sponsored by Go Grains Health and Nutrition Ltd. I am fully aware whilst writing about the benefits of brown rice, dark bread and lentils, that personally I'm not that keen on eating any of these foods and I suspect I'm not the only one. Some of the less scary ways of getting more wholegrain, if the thought of a plate of lentils accompanied by dark bread is not something you can contemplate, are - Shredded Wheat, Fruitful, Cheerios, Muesli, Porridge and homemade popcorn.

I think German eating habits are not exactly the same as those in other countries so I'm not sure it is directly applicable, but a study of over 17,000 Germans by Mandy Schulz (German Institute of Human Nutrition) found that the best predictor of weight loss in women over a two year period was the consumption of cereals. In this case, "cereals" included pasta, cereals, rice, cornflakes and muesli and not specifically just whole grain. (The biggest predictor of weight gain in German women was eating fats, sauces and meat, or in German men, eating more sweets.)

Some other diets - is there any advantage to monounsaturated/omega 3 fats? What about minerals such as calcium, potassium or magnesium? Is green tea any good? Or would you like a diet based on fruit?

Monounsaturated fats and omega-3 fats might have some health benefits but I can find no evidence that they specifically help with weight loss. Similarly, there have been suggestions that certain minerals such as calcium, potassium or magnesium might help with weight loss, but again there has not been any convincing evidence produced.

What about green tea? There has been speculation that green tea helps with weight loss. It contains a mixture of chemicals the most active of which is epigallocatechin gallate (EGCG) which has been speculated to reduce fat absorption and increase the body's energy expenditure. It is often given with caffeine which is thought to enhance its effect. Various trials of EGCG have had conflicting results. For instance, one trial gave half its overweight members a drink of green tea catechin with caffeine and the other half of the group just had a drink with caffeine each day. Dr Kevin Maki reported that there was no difference in the total fat mass between the groups at the end of 12 weeks, but there was greater loss of fat in the stomach area in those in the catechin group. Both groups had side effects and one of the catechin group had to be hospitalised due to high blood pressure.

Dr Olivia Phung (University of Connecticut) analysed the data from all the available trials involving green tea in 2010. She concluded that although there is some evidence of a weight reduction with green tea, the effect is so small that any benefit would not be great and more research is needed. A similar review by Rick Hursel (Maastricht University) of the available evidence found that the effect of catechins on weight loss and maintenance is small, particularly in those who generally have a high caffeine intake anyway, and green tea is less effective in the West than in Asia. This last finding might be due to genetic differences or because Westerners drink more coffee.

It seems reasonable to conclude that any effect of green tea on weight would be very small compared to general dietary intake.

Would eating a lot of fruit help with weight loss? It is generally a healthy food but a trial of two different diets, one with 5% of the calories from fruit and one with 15% of the calories from fruit, found no difference in weight loss between the diets.

Reduced energy density eating - low fat foods and lots of fruit and vegetables

This form of weight control focuses on the fact that people tend to eat a constant volume or weight of food regardless of its composition, as long as it's palatable. Reducing the number of calories in the food without reducing its size or weight can often be done without increasing hunger. Dr Barbara Rolls (Pennsylvania State University) suggests that eating food with a lower energy density could be a new strategy for weight loss and would reduce the problem of hunger. Eating food with higher water content, such as lettuce, apple and steak and avoiding that with low water content, such as bacon, butter and oil is the basic premise of this diet. In practice, it involves eating a low fat diet with a lot of added fruit, vegetables and cooked whole grains. It incorporates strategies such as eating soup before a meal. The sort of changes Dr Rolls outline are, for instance, swapping a lunch of cheeseburger and French fries for a low fat, high vegetable meal - such as grilled chicken salad with low calorie dressing, minestrone soup and garlic bread.

Of course, producing this type of diet tends to result in a diet which is in many ways similar to a low fat diet, as fat is the most energy dense nutrient. Advocates of this approach would include food that is rich in water or fibre and some would consider using substitutes that have been developed for fat and sugar in the diet. It may be that diets that focus on reducing the energy density of food, rather than restricting the overall number of calories, could be more successful. Further research would be needed in this area, but it seems likely that the overall diet would not be too different to a low fat diet with extra fruit and vegetables. This type of eating results in a diet of high quality nutritious food, which is also unfortunately quite expensive. For the dieter, it has the advantage that the message is not "eat less" which leaves them feeling hungry, but to eat less high fat food and to eat as much as they like of food that is low energy density - such as fruit and vegetables.

Do diet websites help? How do they compare with conventional diet methods? Should men stick to the online exercise diary and leave the women to the social forums?

Websites that help people to lose weight are a relatively new phenomenon and there are just a handful of studies that have been done into their effectiveness. It seems that sites that just provide information about diet and exercise are of limited help. Those that provide individual record keeping facilities and personalised feedback are of more benefit to the person wanting to lose weight. Those people with a higher "log on" rate tend to lose more weight, possibly because they are more motivated to lose weight.

There are a few studies that have tried to find out whether internet sites are helpful;

- *More weight was lost using "Calorieking.com.au" than was lost without the website help (in Australia) but the difference was not statistically significant.*

- *No difference in weight loss comparing GP care and internet care in the UK.*

- *Nutracheck seems to be more helpful for men who like to exercise or women who use a chat forum, but no comparison group.*

A study of subscribers to the internet diet service Nutracheck was done by Fiona Johnson (University College London) with help from Nutracheck employees. Unfortunately, it was a retrospective study and people's weight was self-recorded, but it is interesting because it included large numbers of people. 3,600 people were included in the study on the basis that they had recorded two or more weights over at least a month of participating on the programme. Nutracheck currently costs £10 ($17) for a month's membership and includes self-help tools for recording diet, exercise and weight progress. It sets a personal calorie target to lose up to 2lbs (0.9kg) a week. There is a database of over 40,000 items of food, so the calorie value of the food in the user's diary can be calculated. There is also an exercise diary that encourages at least 200 calories to be used in extra activity each day, as well as health and nutritional information and online social support.

The results showed that men lost more weight than women (5.6kg/12lbs versus 3.7kg/8lbs) and lost a higher percentage of their body weight. Those using the food diary facility were more likely to lose a significant amount of weight. Interestingly, using the exercise diary was associated with weight loss in men but not women, whereas using the online forums was associated with weight loss in women but not men. The men using the site were relatively heavier than the women when they started off, were less likely to have tried to lose weight in the past and were more likely to have been prompted to lose weight by a health trigger. It is not clear from the report how long it took to lose the weight or how long it stayed off, but Nutracheck are to be commended for publishing their figures. It would be helpful if more companies could follow their lead, and also look at who benefits from which help. It seems, for example, that if you were a very overweight man who had never dieted before, you might particularly benefit from this sort of help - you should be directed to use the exercise diary and not worry too much about using the chat forums.

- *In Canada, "in person dieting help" beats an internet programme.* Comparing an "internet programme" with an "internet programme with once a month in person meetings" to "only in person help" was done in a study in Vermont of nearly 500 people by Jean Harvey-Berino. After 6 months, the "in-person only" group had lost more weight, at 8kg (18lbs), compared to 5.5kg (12lbs) for the "internet only" group and 6kg (13lbs) for the group that had "internet plus once a month meetings".

As you can see, due to the limited amount of research done on the use of web based diet help, it is not possible to come to any firm conclusions as to how effective they are, or whether they help maintain weight loss. People tend to log on more often when there is counsellor support, support from other dieters, email contact and updates to the website. There are indications that logging on more frequently is more likely to be associated with weight loss. It seems that the more successful sites are those that allow the clients to tailor the programme to suit their own needs.

I did notice when looking at some of these websites, that many of them suggest that you put your height and weight into a box that then calculates your BMI. They then ask how much weight you want to lose and let you set a goal weight. For instance, on one site you can put in that you are a 40 year old woman, 5 ft 4 inches tall, who weighs 9 stone 7lbs (60kg/132lbs) and it will allow you to set a goal weight of 7 stone 10lbs (49kg/108lbs). This is right at the lower end of the healthy weight band of BMI. I think it is questionable whether anyone wants to be at a weight that bordering on underweight. If you do set a goal weight, it's just my opinion, but I think no less than the middle of the healthy weight band for your height might be much more appropriate.

Healthy low fat foods or calorie restriction?

Having a diet that is calorie restricted might produce initial weight loss but people find these diets difficult to stick to because they get hungry, and their body may adapt its metabolism to oppose weight change. There is also the work involved in continually monitoring what you are eating in the form of calorie counting and weighing food, which makes long term adherence to a diet less likely. There is now some interest in *Ad Libitum* diets for weight loss, where the dieter can eat as much as they like of food that is healthy, for instance by sticking to food that is lower in fat. This gets around the problem of feeling so restricted and hungry. Once the dieter recognises what they can eat they do not feel so deprived and the amount of monitoring is less than with counting calories. There may be other advantages; for instance, those on an unlimited low fat diet tend to eat more fruit, vegetables and dairy foods than those on a calorie controlled diet, leading to higher vitamin C and calcium levels.

Is just eating healthy low fat food as good as restricting calories when it comes to weight loss? There is a lack of definitive research into this question. However, the CARMEN (Carbohydrate Ratio Management in European National Diets) trial of nearly 400 obese adults by Professor W. Saris (Maastricht University) compared weight loss in people who were put on a low fat diet where they could eat as much as they wanted, with control groups on normal diet. There were 3 groups;

- Group 1 - eat as much as they like of low fat foods with high simple carbohydrates (such as sugar, syrup and fruit) Lost 0.9kg(2lbs) in six months.
- Group 2 - eat as much as they like of low fat foods with high complex carbohydrates (such as bread, pasta, oatmeal, rice, broccoli and legumes). Lost 1.8kg(4lbs) in six months.
- Group 3 - Their normal food - gained weight (of around 1kg/2.2lbs).

Complex carbohydrates are generally healthier and take longer to digest than simple carbohydrates. These two types of carbohydrates (complex and simple) were looked at because in some countries eating more "low fat food" has been associated with increased obesity (the American Paradox). This may be because many of the foods manufactured and claiming to be "low fat" have a lot of sugar to replace the fat, and are then just as high in calories as the original high fat version. Group 1 were including these sorts of products, whereas group 2 were eating healthier unrefined foods.

From this study, if you want to control weight by eating as much as you like of low fat food, then you should be eating the carbohydrate part of the diet in the form of foods such as vegetables, oatmeal, pasta, bread etc - and not so much of the sugary or syrupy type of low fat food. More weight will be lost eating the naturally low fat vegetables, pasta etc than eating desserts labelled as "low fat" that have a lot of sugar.

This method of eating would mean that you were eating as much as you liked, until you were no longer hungry, of most vegetables, pasta, bread, lean meat, lean chicken and fish etc, cooked without any significant addition of fat. On average, the loss of weight will be fairly small and tend to plateau after about four months, but it does seem that you will be unlikely to put weight on.

Unfortunately, this trial only lasted six months - it would have been interesting to see the results for a longer period.

What is best for you?

"Diets do not work" is a commonly held belief. In fact, the general evidence seems to be that diets do lead to weight loss which is most marked after about six months and is often followed by some regain of weight as time goes on. The evidence generally about diets is poor because of the difficulty of accurately recording what people are eating over a long period of time, and of getting them to stick to changes in diet for any length of time. There is certainly no "magic diet" that is easy to follow and will cause the majority of larger people to lose weight and keep it off. The term dieting is so vague and the effect on the individual so variable that it is impossible to be definitive on the effectiveness of dieting as a whole.

I think it is important to see what is on offer because later in this book we will discuss how the individual will lose weight. People who do lose weight successfully and keep it off often adapt diet regimes to their own lifestyles - it is the individual approach that seems the way forward. Don't make any decisions now - read the rest of the book and later chapters will help you work out what you might do to address any weight problem. As long as you are getting a balanced nutritional diet, then modifying your eating in a way that suits you and is sustainable, is probably the most effective way of keeping weight off in the long term.

In talking about diet it is worth being aware of the "Last Supper Effect". This was demonstrated by Dr Dax Urbszat (University of Toronto) who told a group of female students that they were going to participate in a study of food deprivation and taste perception. Half of the women were told (falsely) that they would start a seven day diet once they had tasted some cookies (which would not be allowed on the diet). The rest of the women were not expecting to diet. Each woman was then left alone with three plates of cookies to taste over ten minutes and was told to help herself as, "We have tons." Among the women who were generally not restrained in their eating patterns, they ate the same amount of cookies whether they thought they were about to start a diet or not. However, for the women who were generally restrained eaters (tended to watch what they ate to avoid gaining or to lose weight) - those who thought they were about to diet ate considerably more cookies than those who were not expecting to diet. If you are contemplating a diet on which you might feel deprived, it might well lead you to eat more in the run up to starting the diet.

Also, all these diets refer to adults. A younger person with a weight problem needs specialist help from a dietician or doctor. Professor G Patton (University of Melbourne) found that among 14 and 15 year old girls, those who were moderate dieters were more likely to develop an eating disorder than their non-dieting school friends. Over a year, their chances of developing an eating disorder were 1 in 40, compared to 1 in 500 for non-dieting girls.

As for the question posed at the beginning of this chapter "does dieting work and if so which is the best?" it seems that dieting does work in the short term of around six months but often fails to deliver the hoped for results long term, when there may be partial or total regain of weight. No one diet stands out as far superior to others and the results for individuals on the same diet or diet plan can vary wildly. Finding a healthy and safe way of coping with food and eating that suits the individual seems to be the way forward, and we shall come back to this with specific steps the individual can take towards the end of this book.

Chapter 4: Exercise - does it help with weight loss?

It is widely accepted that some exercise is good for maintaining the body's health, but does it help with weight loss? Surprisingly, the answer is that it depends on who you are and what your genes are like. If you are the sort of person that is constitutionally predisposed to experience an increase in appetite in response to exercise, then you might get little benefit from extra exercise. Men and women react differently to exercise and being older might also influence whether you lose weight or not.

 Some people will lose much more weight if they take extra exercise and some will lose very little additional weight. This chapter is aimed at helping you to find out which category you are likely to fall into. Should you put on some sports clothes, join a gym and take up mountain biking? Or just go for a short stroll each day?

The more calories the body uses up, the fewer will be left over to make fat tissue, and activity is one of the main ways in which calories are lost. The total number of calories used each day consists of the calories used just to keep the body ticking over at rest, plus those used to digest food, plus the calories used in activity.

For anyone wanting to lose weight, it is not easy to adjust the amount of calories used just to keep the body going. The amount of calories lost as a result of digestion will be dependent on diet, so looking to use more calories in activity is an area that deserves attention.

The alarm activated treadmill

The energy we use in activity consists of that used in playing sport plus that used in non-exercise activity (which is all other activity) such as going to work, shopping, playing the piano, dancing and so forth. Most people do not play sport (65% of adults in England do not play organised weekly sport) so it is this non-exercise activity which is more important. This can vary by as much as 2,000 calories a day between similar sized people, depending on the level of activity in their lifestyle.

Taking this information at face value has led to a trend to advocate an intensive exercise programme for anyone with a weight problem. Whilst the intention might be good, whether this is the best approach for the individual is questionable. For instance, Dr James Levine (Mayo Clinic, Minnesota) has come up with some ways in which people can increase the amount of non-exercise activity they take. These ideas include decorating the spare room in the evening, when they come home from work. This increases the calories used from around 30 (if just sitting in front of the TV) to around 1,000 for an evening's decorating.

He also suggests the television could be moved out of the living room (I'm not sure where to) and that the office day could start with a group yoga session. School buses could drop the children off a mile from the school. In the classroom, the desks could have a treadmill device, or teachers could teach whilst the students shoot basketball hoops. Other ideas that he has come up with include the alarm clock that could also start a bedroom treadmill, or the TV designed only to operate when a treadmill is in use (assuming you have found the TV after moving it out of the lounge).

In support of these types of measures he has studied volunteers who have been banned from using machinery in their daily life. He found that washing up by hand uses up 1.8 calories per minute, compared to 1.3 calories per minute when using a dishwasher (although the volunteers using the dishwasher just loaded it and then watched television). Similarly, he found more calories were used hand washing than by machine, walking to work rather than driving and taking the stairs as opposed to taking the lift. Although not advocating the abolition of all labour saving devices, he then calculates that not using such machinery would lead to the use of enough extra calories to lose about 10lb (4.5kg) of weight each year.

Personally, I would not want to be woken up by an alarm activated treadmill. Nor would I think it wise, at my age, to get on it without any preamble such as a cup of tea or breakfast. If I then had to walk to an office and take the stairs to be greeted by a group yoga session, I'm not sure it would cause me to use up any more calories. If I had to do all this, the chances are I would be exhausted and not move from a chair for the rest of the day. This would then lower my energy expenditure considerably. I might also struggle to decorate the spare room in the evening, after walking home from work. Also, many people either do not want or need to lose weight, or are underweight, yet these suggestions seem to be aimed at the general population. If a child is underweight, then making them walk an extra mile to school and use a treadmill desk is going to be singularly unhelpful. The alternative is just to pick out the larger students to have a treadmill and that would be awful.

Dr Levine did some further interesting experiments that suggest that generally getting up and walking about more could have a positive effect on weight problems. For 10 days he monitored 10 lean and 12 obese volunteers, who all had sedentary jobs, to see how much they walked in their normal life. They all had around 50 short walks a day, each less than 15 minutes duration and at speeds of about 1mph. The lean people walked about 10 miles a day - more than the obese people, who averaged 7 miles. The walking bouts in the larger people tended to be shorter.

He then overfed all the volunteers by an extra 1,000 calories a day, for 8 weeks. This seems quite an undertaking for the volunteers. Measurements at the end of this time showed all the people had put on weight (averaging 3.6kg/8lbs) and they all reduced their walking distance by 1.5 miles a day. For all of the volunteers, there was a correlation between walking distance and body fat. He concluded that walking is reduced in obesity and declines as weight is gained. The implication is that spending less time sitting and more walking, might help with a weight problem. (Or, I wonder if it could be that being larger makes it more difficult to move, so people tend to move less, rather than the lack of movement being the cause of the weight problem? Perhaps it's a bit of both?) Obese people tend to sit for 2.5 hours a day more than people who are of lean build.

In any case, getting up and walking more about the office or going for a stroll in the lunch hour, seems to me more acceptable than having a treadmill attached to the desk. Trying to make blanket generalisations about the amount of activity that is beneficial to people is not very practical and probably the best way forward is to treat people as individuals.

There is some debate about the effect of exercise on weight. Studying this is difficult, as getting larger people to take monitored exercise for any length of time is not easy. Unfortunately, many of the tests involve small groups of people for relatively short time periods. Testing for the effect of exercise is often done by introducing extra exercise sessions such as cycling, or treadmill use, as it is easier to quantify the effects compared to just increasing activity generally.

Women eat more with exercise

Men and women seem to react differently to exercise and most studies indicate that vigorous exercise reduces the amount that men subsequently go on to eat (although one study found there was little difference in the amount men eat after exercise).

In contrast, women tend to get hungrier after exercise and eat more. Marjorie Pomerleau (University of Ottawa) subjected a small group of women to variable exercise and found that the women ate more. The increased appetite and food consumption would be the equivalent of 25% of the calories used up in exercise when the exercise was low intensity (walking on a treadmill) and just over 40% of the calories when the exercise was high intensity (fast walking on a treadmill). This implies that if you are a woman wanting to lose weight, you might prefer to take lower level exercise rather than strenuous exercise, which will have less relative benefit.

When women take exercise, they get changes in the levels of some of the hormones associated with appetite control (acylated ghrelin goes up and insulin levels are lower). These changes stimulate appetite and cause eating. It is thought that these changes are helping the body to try and match the calories eaten with those used up in exercise, as the body tries to maintain its weight. Women, in general, eat more to replace all or some of the lost calories. This is likely to be because the female body is designed to preserve its fat stores for reproduction. Women are meant to be "curvy" and it is known that not eating enough can reduce fertility. The changes in women's hormones are therefore probably a protective mechanism to ensure that they do not get too thin. Unfortunately, this makes it more difficult for women to lose weight than men.

In men, there is no effect of exercise alone on these regulatory hormones. Men lose body fat when exercising and eating what they want (ad libitum feeding) but women tend not to.

Some people compensate for exercise by eating more - there is a huge variation in the extent of this effect

There is some variability in the amount the appetite increases with exercise (in addition to the gender effect described above). This partial compensation to replace some of the calories used in exercise has led researchers to categorise people as either "compensators" who eat more with exercise, or "non-compensators" who do not. There is a suggestion that among compensators the effect of exercise is to increase the pleasure of eating and that this does not occur in non-compensators.

Dr Graham Findlayson (University of Leeds) looked at the appetite of a small group of women by monitoring how much they ate of a meal, on one occasion, when they had not been exercising, and on another occasion when they had been cycling for nearly an hour. Some of the women ate more after exercise. These compensator women rated food as more palatable after exercise and also showed a preference for high fat sweet food, whether they had exercised or not, when compared to the non-compensators.

Dr Findlayson went on to do further tests, this time with sedentary men and women whose weight category was obese. They agreed to exercise by cycling 5 days a week, using an extra 500 calories each exercise session. He found that the non-compensators lost around 5kg (11lbs) of fat and the compensators lost an average of 2kg (4.4lbs) of fat, over the 3 month trial. Again, he found that the liking for food increased in the compensators after exercise and they showed the same preference for high fat sweet food. However, by the end of the trial, although they still liked and wanted food after exercise, there was no longer the preference for high fat sweet food. It seems that exercise over a period of a few months can cause taste to change, so that food that is healthier, lower in fat and less likely to contribute to a weight problem becomes more preferable.

Men and women with a BMI of around 32 (moderately obese) were the subject of a study into the effect of exercise by Prof. Neil King (University of Leeds). This was interesting as it also involved people with a significant weight problem. This group of 35 people (average age 40 years) exercised 5 times a week in supervised conditions for 3 months. Again, there seemed to be a difference between those who compensated for exercise by eating more and those who did not.

The compensators lost an average of 1.5kg (3.3lbs) of weight, were hungrier on the programme and ate an additional 268 calories per day. Their metabolic rate reduced by a small amount (60kcal/day) but this was not a big enough drop to be statistically different to any change in the metabolic rate of the non-compensators, which stayed about the same. Despite doing all the exercise, some of these people actually gained weight. On the other hand, the non-compensators lost an average of 6.3kg (14lbs) and they ate less, did not report any appetite change and the amount they were eating each day decreased by an average of 130 calories.

There was a huge amount of individual variation in the response to exercise. The research indicates that this is less due to the change in metabolism of the compensators, but more due to changes in the behaviour of these exercisers. This could be due to increased eating in response to exercise. Whilst some of this is under conscious control (such as buying a doughnut on the way home from the gym) some could be automatic subconscious behaviour (such as increasing the portion size of the next meal). It has been suggested that as well as satisfying hunger, food might be seen as a "reward" and this response sensitivity to reward could possibly be a character trait.

These types of prescribed exercise sessions (similar to going to the gym) will help some people with weight loss but there is a great amount of individual variation. Those people who do not compensate for exercise by eating more may well lose weight but the compensators will eat more, initially showing a preference for high fat food which if they continue for a few months might well change to a preference for less fatty, healthier food. The reasons that these compensators lose less weight or put weight on with exercise include:

- Increased hunger and eating more.
- Perhaps being less active in the non-exercising part of the day as they are tired from the exercise.
- Having a small reduction in metabolic rate as a result of the weight loss.

There does seem to be a big individual variation in the effect of exercise on weight. Probably the categorisation of people into compensators and non-compensators is an arbitrary decision as to where to "draw a line in the sand" as it were, and is a helpful research tool. In practice, some people might clearly fall into one category or the other, whereas others might be more borderline cases. At the end of this chapter there will be a discussion about how this information can relate to you, as an individual.

Even those in the "compensator" category still need exercise for health

Unfortunately, there is no widely available test to take to find out whether you are a compensator or non-compensator and even most of the compensators lose a small amount of weight on average with exercise. If you fall into the compensator category, it does not mean you should not move at all, because it is necessary to have some activity for health reasons. If you think you are in the compensator category it might be a better use of your time to go for a walk each day, if you want to lose weight, rather than head off for an exhausting session at the gym. There is also the possible benefit that you might find low fat healthy food more appealing with regular exercise.

Low fat food tastes better with regular exercise

Women in Leeds who were described as "restrained eaters" (they tended to restrict their food intake to prevent weight gain) were offered a buffet lunch after either a period of rest or a 50 minute cycling session. Two sorts of lunch were tested - one was high fat, consisting of sandwiches, coleslaw, crisps, quiche, chocolate biscuits, Viennese whirls and fruit fool. The other lunch was a low fat buffet of sandwiches, coleslaw, breadsticks, pizza, jaffa cakes, swiss-roll and fruit yoghurt. This small group of women did not become hungrier after exercise and they ate nearly 70% more calories when offered the high fat buffet, than when offered the low fat buffet, regardless of whether they had been exercising or not. The weight of food was the same but it was more calorie dense when high fat. The low fat buffet was rated as more pleasant after they had been exercising. The researcher, Dr Anne Lluch (University of Leeds) thought it was possible that a low fat diet, when combined with exercise, could help prevent obesity, as these results suggest that exercise might help people get more pleasure from food that is lower in fat.

The same breakfast is more "filling" if you're taking regular exercise

A larger study of overweight or obese middle-aged men and women was done by Prof. Neil King (Queensland University). It looked at whether taking exercise could make meals feel more filling. These people agreed to undertake 3 months of supervised exercise, such as on a treadmill or cycling machine, for 5 days each week. On the day of the exercise, the participants were fed a fixed breakfast of cereal, milk, toast, margarine, jam and tea with milk. The amount was decided by how much they ate at the initial session and the average calorie content was 400 calories.

It was found that the reduction in body weight was very variable, with the non-compensators having no increase in hunger, losing an average of 15% of their total body fat and reducing their daily calorie intake by 126kcal. In contrast, the compensators lost an average of 5% of their body weight and ate an extra 164kcal/day and were significantly hungrier before breakfast.

All the exercisers found the fixed breakfast significantly more filling towards the end of the programme, leading to the conclusion that exercise can affect the appetite in two ways; it leads some people to get hungry and eat more and it also increases the filling effect of a meal. It is though, I think, possible that the fixed breakfast seemed more filling because it was in fact "fixed" and we know that the desire to eat can be influenced by variety. Maybe the participants grew weary of eating the same breakfast over and over again, leading them to rate it as more filling? Whatever the mechanism, the identical breakfast caused a greater immediate reduction in hunger, which lasted until just before lunch.

Could regular exercise help you to tell the difference between a high calorie milkshake loaded with cream and a regular shake?

A group of normal weight men were invited to the University of Surrey, by Prof. Linda Morgan, where they were each given a milkshake at 11.30am. Two different milkshakes had been prepared using ingredients such as double cream and sugars - one drink was made up to contain 240 kcal and the other contained 600 kcal. The participants were not told of the difference and were randomly allocated either the high or low calorie drink. An hour later, a buffet lunch was served, where what they ate was monitored.

It was found that the men who normally took regular exercise in their lives significantly reduced how much they ate at the buffet when they had drunk the high calorie drink, compared to when they had had the low calorie drink. The men who did not habitually take exercise did not modify their consumption at all with the high calorie drink and there was no significant decline in their food consumption. This implies that exercise might help sharpen up the appetite response to food - either that or those who are disposed to take regular exercise also tend to have better capacity to know when they have eaten enough and to stop eating. Of those who did take regular exercise, those that took moderate levels of exercise were better at regulating their appetite than those who took particularly vigorous exercise.

Genes influence sport

There is evidence that there is a genetic effect on the amount of sporting type exercise we participate in and on our activity levels generally.

I am always quite bemused as to why people feel the need to run marathons, for instance, when there is a perfectly adequate bus system. The thought of running that distance holds no appeal to me at all. Perhaps these people are responding in part to some genetic predisposition to exercise? Certainly, they don't seem to be running for the health benefits. Yearly injury rates for those training for marathons have been reported to be as high as 90%. Those at especially high risk of injury are the less experienced runners training over 40 miles a week. Effects of actually running the marathon can include injuries to the knees, as well as leg and feet injuries, muscle soreness, blisters, chaffing, abrasions, malaise, stomach upsets, exhaustion, nausea and chills. Yet many people take part in these running events in what seems to me to be a huge demonstration of wasted energy - if they have that much spare energy couldn't they mow a lawn or plant a tree or something? It is likely, I think, that my genetic pool lacks any of the genes which predispose to exercise.

There is good evidence that a tendency to take part in sport is inherited. A study that used data from thousands of twins was analysed by Dr Janine Stubbe (Vrije University). She found that participating or not in exercise activities in leisure time has a genetic component. Data from nearly 40,000 pairs of twins from many countries was analysed. Whilst men consistently reported slightly greater exercise participation than women, the resemblance of exercise participation in identical twins was higher than in non-identical twins and the results were consistent with a genetic influence on sports participation. The influence of genetics on exercise behaviour varied from country to country - for instance, in women aged 19-40 years in the UK, genetic influences accounted for 70% in the variation in their exercise behaviour (the rest is due to environmental factors).

Other research shows that this genetic influence on sport does not kick in until after the age of 15 years, as before this age a child's activities are largely out of its control and decided by parents and teachers. However, by the time the age of 20 is reached, genetics are deciding how much sport is played, with the heritability of exercise participation shooting up from zero at the age of 15, to reach 80% at the age of 20. "Heritability" of the tendency to play sport or not, is the proportion of the differences in sports playing behaviour between people in the population, that is caused by differences in their genes.

This means 80% is the difference in exercise behaviour between people aged 20 that is due to genetic differences. It then starts to fall fairly rapidly, so by the time the age of 30 is reached, the heritability is 50%. If you have inherited the genes that predispose you to participate in exercise, then you are likely to find yourself playing sport in your late teens.

Although a heritability of 80% implies that much voluntary exercise is genetically determined, that proportion is not fixed. For instance, if the environment were to change, then it could play a bigger part in whether people were exercising or not than it currently does, and the influence of genetics would be lessened. If, for instance, everyone had their TV's removed and they were provided with swimming pools and tennis courts at home, then this environmental change would be likely to affect the amount of exercise being done. The genetic contribution to exercise might be smaller and the environmental contribution larger. This sort of factor might be contributing to the difference in heritability of sporting behaviour between countries. In Australia, the influence of genetic factors on exercise is around 50%, compared to the UK where the genetic factors account for around 70% of the variation in sporting activity. The environmental facilities for sport seem to make more of a difference in whether sport is played in Australia.

These studies imply that for the individual, whether they take part in sporting type exercise or not around the age of 20 will be largely influenced by the genes they have inherited - as they age this influence of inheritance diminishes.

What decides whether we play sport or are an armchair spectator?

If you have a mother who is a marathon runner in the Olympics and a father who is an international footballer, then you are likely to have inherited an athletic build. This will make you more likely to be good at sport and the positive praise you get for your achievements will encourage you to continue participating. If you are athletic, you have largely inherited your build and responsiveness to training, which will make you more likely to continue in sport. Body shape, size, muscular strength, flexibility and speed, all have a large inherited component. People tend to do what they are good at and if you excel at sport you are more likely to continue participating.

On the other hand, if you come from a family whose body shape is generally stocky, with no sporting talent and no matter how hard you try, you never get picked for the football team, then you are less likely to continue with sport. You are more likely to focus on other areas of life when finding an achievement at which you can excel.

As well as body size and shape, it is also possible that genes could influence mood after exercise and determine whether it is one of exhilaration or exhaustion. If you feel good after exercise, you are probably more likely to repeat the experience than if you just feel exhausted.

Whilst the most common reason that women give for participating in exercise is "to lose weight", the most common reason for men is "to stay in shape". Genes that predispose to fitness might influence men to exercise.

Genes have also been shown to have an effect on our personalities and some researchers have speculated that factors such as self-motivation might increase the tendency to participate in sports. Other factors, such as poor self-esteem, might reduce the likelihood of participation. I can find no evidence to support this view. There is, however, some evidence that those whose personalities tend slightly more to extravert and "sensation seeking" are more likely to seek out exercise.

As people get older, recreational exercise is more common than competitive sport and at this stage the genes influencing personality might become more influential. A large study of twins in the Netherlands (also by Dr Stubbe) found that, on average, exercisers have slight tendencies to be more extravert and sensation seeking and slightly less anxious, depressed or neurotic than non-exercisers. This seems to be a personality trait causing people to seek out exercise if they are extravert and less anxious, depressed or neurotic, rather than the exercise making them feel less anxious and so forth.

As well as sporting type exercise, there is also a significant genetic effect on the habitual level of physical activity - that is, the other non-sporting activity that forms part of our daily lives. Annemiek Joosen (Maastricht University) measured the energy expenditure in identical and non-identical twins and found that there was a high genetic contribution to the variation in physical activity in daily life. It seems that our genes influence how active we are in normal life, as well as whether we play sport.

Although research is going on to find the genes which influence our level of activity, and potential genes have been identified, there is still a long way to go. Physical activity is probably determined by multiple genes as well as factors in the environment. For the moment, trying to work out whether you have a sporting disposition or not (or indeed a tendency to compensate for exercise by eating more) is probably best done by considering your own experience and physique and that of your close relatives. In the future, further developments might make it possible to devise individual strategies for weight problems based on genetic predisposition.

Why do men play more sport than women?

As for the tendency for men to be slightly more sporting than women, some of this might be attributable to men thinking they get more benefit from exercise. The most common reason given by men for exercising is "to stay in shape" whereas for women it is "to lose weight" (although exercise might be more helpful for men in weight loss). However, in my opinion, some of the discrepancy in sport participation may well be due to the widespread discrimination against female sport in favour of male sport.

Take football - in England this was a very popular female sport attracting large crowds of spectators, until it was banned in the 1920's by the England Football Association (FA). They voted that no woman should play using any of its club facilities. This ban was not cancelled until the 1970's, when even the men of the FA could not hold out against some gesture towards equality. It does seem to have been little more than a gesture however, as the current FA Women's Cup Final is being held not at Wembley, where many people might have actually gone to see it, but in Doncaster. Similarly, the proportion of sports reporters and match commentators that are female is generally reported as being less than 10%, and might be nearer 3%.

The message for women in the UK is clear - sport is for men. This is reinforced by television coverage of sport, which overwhelmingly features men. Given that half the population is female and there is no reduction in paying the TV licence for women, perhaps the BBC (state run television company) should be required to broadcast the same amount of sports coverage featuring women's sport as men's sport, at an equivalent time of day. This probably will not happen, because although we now have the legislation for equality, in practice most establishments pay lip service to this, whilst continuing to discriminate shamefully. Twice as many men than women hold senior roles in the BBC and they are paid an average of £17,000 more than the women.

Private versus state schools?

In children, when both parents are active, the child is nearly six times as likely to be active than the child of two sedentary parents. This is presumably because the parents might get the child to join them in sport, they act as role models and are themselves genetically predisposed to physical activity. Children do not get much personal choice about how much they play sport because it is largely out of their control and depends on local facilities and parental influence.

Dr Katie Mallam (Plymouth University) compared children in England at a private preparatory school who did 9 hours of PE each week, with children at an inner city state school who did 1.8 hours of PE a week. She asked the children, who were aged nine, to wear accelerometers (movement detecting devices). It was found that there was little difference in the total activity of the children between schools. The state school children were much more active outside school hours. Possibly the privately educated children did not have as much energy left to be active after all the PE.

Exercise when older

Particularly in the older age group, the part played by sport in activity levels is generally small and does not have much effect on total energy (calorie) requirements. Most of the difference in calorie use between people, is due to difference in the levels of spontaneous activity and not due to sport or prescribed exercise.

Michael Goran (University of Vermont) subjected eleven healthy people aged 56-68 to a programme of endurance training over 8 weeks. They attended cycling sessions 3 times a week, building up to a total of 3 hours a week. He calculated that their increase in energy expenditure was the equivalent of 150 calories per day. There was also an increase in their resting metabolic rate, equivalent to 167 calories per day. However, there was no increase at all in the total number of calories these people were using up, despite all their hard work cycling. The reason was that there was a significant reduction in the amount of activity that these people could undertake for the rest of the day, once they had finished the cycling. So, if you are in your late fifties and are considering cycling for an hour a day 3 times a week, you may end up using no more calories than if you had not bothered - if, after cycling, you are so tired that you come home, collapse in a chair and do not move for the rest of the day. However, there was an improvement in the cardiovascular fitness of the volunteers - so although they did not use more calories, they did at least get fitter.

Men benefit more from exercise

Not surprisingly, if you are taking part in endurance training in order to run a half marathon, your physical activity levels (as measured by wearing an accelerometer to detect movement) will go up. Dr Gerwin Meijer (Netherlands) monitored a small group of people age 28-41 years, as they trained over five months. He found that their physical activity increased by 60% by the end of the training period. In women, physical activity did not change in the non-training part of the day, but in men there was a slight increase (15%), and their average daily metabolic rate increased significantly. It seems that in men, exercise tends to increase other physical activity and also diet induced thermogenesis (more calories are used in food digestion), but these effects do not occur in women. This suggests that women get slightly less benefit from endurance training than men, if they are trying to lose weight.

This is not to say that if you are a man trying to lose weight, running a half marathon is the best way to go about it. Do check with your doctor before signing up for any such event. I remember when I was working in coronary care, seeing a middle-aged man who was admitted to hospital with a heart attack at the end of a half marathon. Although the nurse warned me that he was livid, I was surprised to find he was indeed the most notably angry patient I had ever admitted. Although I had never seen him before in my life, so could not be in any way responsible for his condition, I had to keep reminding myself that I was not really the target of his anger. I suppose it is understandable that if you think that such an activity is beneficial to health and you find instead that it can be so detrimental, you might indeed be somewhat irritated. Later in this book will be advice on how the individual can cope with a weight problem, but perhaps I should say here that once you get to middle-age it is, in my opinion, generally much safer to take up sports such as golf, gentle swimming or walking (as opposed to squash or marathon running), should you wish to take additional exercise.

Exercise though, does seem to have some advantage for men trying to lose weight. Barbara Frey-Hewitt (Stanford University) monitored 120 overweight sedentary men over a period of one year. Forty of the men followed a diet, 40 took exercise by jogging 10 miles each week, and the rest neither dieted nor exercised. At the end of the year, both the diet group and the exercise group had lost a significant amount of weight compared to the control group, who had no change in their weight. However, the diet group had a small but significant drop in their resting metabolic rate (their bodies were using up less calories) compared to the exercise group or the control group. This does seem to support the case for doing some exercise if you are male and have a weight problem.

Would exercising for 45 minutes a day, 5 days a week without dieting appeal to you as a method of weight loss? Joseph Donnelly (University of Kansas) got nearly 90 overweight or moderately obese men and women to do this. Only around half of them managed to keep up the exercise until the end of the 16 month trial. The people were all aged 17-35 years and had a sedentary lifestyle prior to the experiment, which mostly involved supervised treadmill walking, in a research environment. At the end of the trial, the men had lost 5kg (11lbs) and the women had lost no weight, which seems to reinforce the case for exercise being more helpful for men than women. There was, however, a control group who did no exercise and the female controls put on an average of 3kg (6.6lbs). Although the exercising women did not lose any weight, exercise at least seemed to help them prevent more weight accumulating.

Women might get less weight loss from exercise but does moving about more in daily life stop weight gain?

Measuring the amount of physical activity that people undertake in normal daily living can now be done by finding how much energy they are using, without them having to record activities, by using a technique involving doubly labelled water. People drink water which has been made up from water molecules containing naturally occurring variations on the normal oxygen and hydrogen atoms. The rate at which they are excreted from the body is measured over a period of about a fortnight. This, when taken with a measure of their basal metabolic rate, can be used to calculate the level of physical activity in normal life.

Sixty women who had a sedentary lifestyle and did not take regular exercise were monitored for a year (by Dr Roland Weinsier, University of Alabama) to see which of them put on weight, and whether there was a relationship between general activity and weight gain. The women were all a normal weight at the beginning of the year but around half of them had previously had to lose weight in order to get to a normal weight. At the end of the year, it was found that most of those who had put on weight were from the group that had been previously overweight, and those that had gained weight had had a lower level of physical activity than the others. It was calculated that this lower level in itself was enough to account for nearly 80% of the weight gain. This suggests that for women, particularly those with a previous weight problem, generally increasing activity levels (such as by walking, taking the stairs and undertaking activities such as gardening) might be helpful in preventing weight gain.

Walking is as good as jogging in middle-age? Walking an additional six miles a week might be enough to stop weight going up

Perhaps the level of exercise needed to stop weight gain is not too extreme? Dr C Slentz (Duke University) compared the effect of jogging 20 miles, jogging 12 miles, or walking 12 miles each week, using over 100 overweight sedentary men and women in the age group 40-65 years. The volunteers were told not to change the type or quantity of food that they normally ate and were encouraged not to change their weight, so that just the effect of exercise over the 8 month trial was considered. A control group who did not exercise put on over 2kg (4.4lbs) but the exercisers all lost weight, more so in the group that were doing the most vigorous exercise (4.8kg/10.6lbs fat mass lost). However, there was not much difference between the groups that were jogging 12 miles (2.5kg/5.5lbs fat lost) or walking (2kg/4.4lbs fat lost). Once again, the weight loss was less for women than for men, but in this case there was little difference when it was expressed as a percentage change in body weight.

It seems a minimal amount of physical activity is needed to stop weight increasing (as the non-exercisers put on weight). From this study, it was calculated that the average amount needed might be as little as walking 6 extra miles a week, to prevent weight gain in someone who is overweight and sedentary.

Taking exercise while dieting can mean more of the weight lost consists of fat compared to weight lost by just dieting

In a small study, 8 obese women were admitted to hospital where for 5 weeks they only consumed 800 calories each day, as a vanilla or chocolate flavoured liquid diet. Some of the women also participated in an exercise regime that involved walking with a member of staff each day, gradually increasing the distance. The average amount of weight lost was the same whether the women walked or not (8kg/18lbs) but of the women that had the daily walk, 74% of the weight lost was fat tissue compared to 57% in the non-walking women. The resting metabolic rate declined around 20% in both groups, but the researcher (James Hill, Vanderbilt University) reported that there was an indication that the effect of exercise might be to slightly attenuate the expected fall in metabolic rate.

The implications are that if you're dieting to lose weight, taking a daily walk might mean that a greater proportion of weight loss is from body fat. You might, perhaps, also avoid some of the unhelpful reduction in metabolic rate that can occur when on a diet.

Diet versus diet plus exercise

There are many studies into the effects of exercise and diet on weight. There is a problem in that they often limit themselves to studying only either men or women. In addition, the level of excess weight seems to be on the low side when experiments are done which require getting larger people to exercise. There is also a tendency to report average weight loss, instead of how many people actually lose weight, which is more relevant.

Sometimes researchers seem to be a little naïve - one study I read stated that the participants were instructed by a dietician to eat only 800 calories each day for 16 weeks and monitoring was by periodic interview and self-kept reports. It would be very difficult to stick to that small amount of food for such a time period and the temptation would have been huge to omit food from the record, giving much less credibility to the results. It also seems quite difficult to get people at the larger end of the weight spectrum to take part in these sorts of studies - so many seem to focus on people whose weight problem is at the lesser end of the excess weight spectrum.

A review was done in 2005 of all the good trials comparing diet and exercise to diet alone (by Dr C. Curoni, University of Rio de Janeiro). It was found that diet with exercise produced greater weight loss than diet alone in overweight and obese people, both soon after the programmes started and after one year of follow up. However, in both cases there was a weight regain of around 50% at the end of one year and it appeared that the more weight was lost initially, the more difficult it was to avoid regaining weight.

Another review of around 500 studies that used "diet", "exercise" or "diet plus exercise" for weight loss was done in 1997 by Dr W Miller (George Washington University). It was noted that most of the research seemed again to focus more on women than men, who were often only moderately obese and around the age of forty. Many trials were of short duration and particularly with relation to exercise, were conducted on people who were only just in the obese category. Despite these reservations, the analysis concluded that weight loss under the different regimes was:

- Diet alone - around 11kg (24lbs) loss, and after one year 56% of the weight loss was maintained.
- Exercise alone - 3kg (6.6lbs) loss, and after one year 53% of the weight loss was maintained.
- Diet plus exercise -11kg (24lbs) loss, and after one year 77% of the weight loss was maintained.

As you can see, there was some weak evidence that after one year "diet plus exercise" was most effective in keeping weight off.

Is it possible to give a blanket level of exercise that everyone should do?

Efforts to find a level of exercise that suits everyone have not been successful. Prof. John Blundell (University of Leeds) reported the efforts of one of his colleagues to get normal weight and overweight women to do the level of exercise recommended by the World Health Organization (WHO).

In 1990, the WHO recommended an exercise level for benefits to health, wellbeing and fitness. This was aerobic activity for at least 20 minutes, 3-5 times a week, at a level between 50%-85% of the maximum oxygen capacity (VO2max). This is a high intensity level of exercise (VO2max is the most amount of oxygen a person can use when exercising at maximal capacity and high intensity is around 70%).

Although the women were on the supervised exercise regime for 4 weeks, there was no discernible change in the women's total daily energy expenditure (they did not use up any more calories) nor was there any change in the amount eaten, weight or energy balance. The women were found to have mis-reported their food intake and were not able to achieve the exercise goals; managing only 70% of the required levels. Anecdotally, this was because the overweight women found this level of exercise too arduous. Although 25 women started the study, only 9 normal weight and 8 overweight women finished to have their results included in this experiment.

Although the intentions of organisations such as the WHO in prescribing levels of exercise were good, it seems that in practice it was not a realistic option, even though these women were being given close monitoring and supervision. In daily life, the chances of them attaining this level of exercise, for instance by going to a gym, might have been even less.

It seems that a general prescription for exercise in overweight women is of little practical value.

Summary - The effect of exercise on weight loss endeavours

There is a huge variation in the individual response to exercise. It is more beneficial to some people than others, depending on whether they get hungry with exercise and eat more to compensate, or not. There is also a gender difference, with men likely to lose more weight than women. Putting on weight is associated with lower activity levels and moving less.

Exercise does have some general benefits for those wanting to lose weight, in that it seems to help the dieter avoid regaining the weight once it has been lost and it makes healthy low fat food more appealing. If a dieter does exercise, more of the weight that is lost will be fat, as opposed to other body tissues such as muscle.

In the elderly, exercise may not use up any more calories if they are too tired to move for the rest of the day after exercising, although they might get fitter.

How much exercise should you actually do?

People react differently to exercise, so it might be better if the exercise was tailored to the individual. Women get more relative benefit from less arduous exercise. Men tend to get more of a weight loss response from exercise, so if their health permits, they might wish to consider slightly more strenuous exercise.

A later chapter in this book will go into more detail about how the individual can take this sort of information and use it to try and lose weight. For now, if you are considering exercise of the sporting type to help lose weight, such as football, jogging, swimming, cycling, squash and so forth, it seems to depend on your general genetic disposition, age and gender whether this will leave you exhilarated, fitter and thinner or in contrast, hungrier, heading for food and too tired to move for the rest of the day.

In years to come, sophisticated genetic and metabolic testing might be available, but for the present you could take a guess at which category you fall into. If you come from a family of honed international athletes and are surrounded by people weightlifting and doing push-ups, you may well have the type of body that might benefit from more strenuous exercise. If you are male, you are likely to lose more weight from exercise than if you are female. If you are elderly, doing strenuous exercise will not reduce your weight much if you are then too tired to move for the rest of the day. If you enjoy sport, you are probably more likely to benefit constitutionally from it, so if you think this sort of exercise will help, find a sport you enjoy that is appropriate for your age and state of health (check with your doctor first) and go for it. It might possibly also have the side effect of sharpening up your appetite response so your preferences might tend more towards lower fat, more healthy food, which can only be helpful.

What if this is not you? What if you are a woman with a weight problem from a non-athletic family who hates any form of sport and is so hungry after, for instance, a short swim, that you find yourself heading for a coffee and doughnut on the way out of the leisure centre? Perhaps you might wish to discount sporting exercise as a way of helping with weight loss. In any case, most of us do not play sport. Instead, a better approach might be to try and incorporate extra movement into the daily life and to do this frequently in a way that becomes a routine, rather than "taking exercise". If you can walk the children the half mile to school and back instead of dropping them off in the car, this would be the equivalent of around 200 miles of extra walking a year, but it is not a long enough walk to make most people feel hungry or exhausted. In an office job, taking a break at lunch time from the desk to walk to the shops, or across the park, each day, can make a considerable difference to the amount of daily activity.

Of course, as well as helping to lose weight or to stop it accumulating, there are health benefits to becoming more active.

Don't make any decisions about exercise now, read the rest of the book and then hopefully you will be in a better position to pull together the changes that will be most helpful to you. If and when you do decide to change the amount of exercise you are doing, check with your family doctor first to make sure that it will suit you and not cause any risk to your health.

Chapter 5: Who manages to keep weight off once they have lost it and what is the secret to maintaining the loss?

The test of a diet or lifestyle change aimed at weight loss is not really how much weight is lost, or how quickly, but how long it stays off. Many celebrities have been made to look a little foolish by going on a diet or exercise regime and successfully losing weight, at the same time publishing a book or DVD advising others how to follow in their footsteps. They are then photographed a year or two later, clearly having regained all or most of their weight.

An actor from a British soap opera brought out a best-selling fitness DVD, saying she had lost 2.5 stone (35lbs/16kg) with this DVD. Unfortunately, just three months later she appeared to have put a considerable amount of weight back on. Similarly, an ex-singer brought out a workout DVD in 2007, saying that it had helped her to lose 4 stone (56lbs/25kg) and get down to a size 10. Four years later, she was telling a national newspaper that she felt, "confident as a size 16". There are numerous other examples - I can't bring myself to name names, as although they are very unlikely to read this book, most people would be embarrassed to be in this situation.

I am sure that at the time these people made the DVDs they

probably did feel that they had solved their weight problem and genuinely thought that they could help others by sharing their methods of weight loss. However, weight has a tendency to go back on. It might be wise, if you are a celebrity with a diet book or exercise DVD, to wait a couple of years before publishing, just to make sure you don't get embarrassed by unflattering photographic comparisons in the press.

Once you have lost weight, you will want to know how to avoid putting it back on again. It is useful to find out how other people have successfully managed to avoid regaining weight.

Three ways to stop weight regain

In America, there is an association for people who have lost at least 30lbs (14kg) and kept it off for at least a year (The National Weight Control Registry). Its 10,000 members have all chosen to join and there are a large proportion of women. Most are college educated and they have lost an average of just over four stone (66lbs/30kg) for five years. Half were overweight as children, most had a family history of excess weight problems and most had unsuccessful weight loss attempts before finally being successful.

Whilst these people have chosen to join the Registry and therefore might not be representative of the total population of successful weight loss maintainers, it is still helpful to look at what seemed to work for them. Dr Rena Wing (Brown University) found that the members of the registry had three behaviours in common: they were physically active, they ate food that was low in fat and high in carbohydrate, and they weighed themselves regularly.

They had a high level of physical activity. Walking was the most popular form of exercise, with most doing quite a considerable amount - the equivalent of one hour each day. Most of the members did not watch much television, with over 60% watching less than 10 hours each week, which might mean they are sitting less and moving more.

There also appears to be a slight preference for weightlifting, with 20% of the women participating in this, as opposed to around 9% in the population as a whole. The statistics do not reveal whether this is light lifting, as might be done with a small set of dumbbells at a gym as part of a fitness programme, or whether it is the sort of weightlifting that you see at the Olympics, with people sweating and straining to lift a bar above their head. I suspect it is the former. I am at a loss to explain why lifting weights, in particular, should help with maintaining weight loss, unless it is coming up statistically as an indicator that these people are also attending gyms. This finding also occurred in a mailed survey of successful weight loss maintainers done by Dr Judy Kruger (University of Waterloo) where 20% of successful weight loss maintainers reported that they lifted weights, compared to 11% of those that put the weight back on.

The food that these successful weight loss maintainers eat is low in fat and high in carbohydrate. Carbohydrate rich foods include cereals, grains, pasta, bread, fruits and vegetables. Sugar, sweets and cakes are also rich in carbohydrate but it is unlikely that these people were eating these, as they also incorporate a lot of fat in their ingredients. On average, they eat around 1,800 calories each day, with about a quarter of these calories coming from fat. They nearly always eat breakfast, usually cereals and fruit, and they eat the same sort of food weekdays and weekends. (Those who were more flexible, such as eating more at weekends, tended to put weight back on again.) They eat an average of 5 meals or snacks each day, have fast food once a week and eat out at restaurants just over twice a week.

Daily or weekly monitoring of their weight was another behaviour that this group of people adopted to help prevent weight regain.

It seems likely that this information would be useful to someone who has lost weight and wants to avoid putting it back on. Of course, the people that join the Registry might be those that find it more difficult to keep weight off and need to be preoccupied with it. Those that lose weight and keep it off more easily might be less inclined to join. The membership was scrutinised by Dr Lorraine Ogden (University of Colorado) who found that four distinct types of people were represented. The largest group was about half the membership - who had a healthy lifestyle, stable weight and were happy with their life. The second largest group (25%) had had a weight problem from childhood, they needed the largest number of strategies to keep the weight off, and they were more likely to feel stressed. Another group (12%) were not overweight as children, lost weight easily at the first attempt and had little trouble keeping it off. The remaining small group were older, had health problems, ate fewer meals and were least likely to exercise. It does seem that losing weight and keeping it off is much easier for some people than for others.

Most members reported that something happened to trigger their successful weight loss. The triggers included the death of a family member from a heart attack, a medical situation and being told by a doctor to lose weight, or the weight reaching an all time high. Sometimes, seeing themselves in a photo or a mirror was the trigger. Anecdotes in the press often describe how people have decided to tackle their weight problem after seeing a photo - when they find they are "bigger than Santa" or wider than the huge snowman that the children have made in the garden.

The members who gained weight had tended to increase their fat consumption, reduced their physical activity levels and were more likely to have had loss of control whilst eating.

The Christmas holiday period is a very difficult time for those who have lost weight. Dr Suzanne Phelan (Brown Medical School) found that even though these people go to greater efforts to make plans to control their eating and maintain their exercise patterns than the rest of the population, 40% of them put on 1kg or more over the holiday period. In the general population who have not had a weight problem, only 17% put on this much weight over the holidays. If you have lost weight, the winter holiday season is a difficult time and it seems you need to be on full alert to avoid the weight going back on.

The good news is that once members had managed to keep the weight off for two years, the subsequent risk of regaining weight was reduced by 50%. Perhaps, after a while, whatever strategies that are being used to maintain the new weight become second nature to some extent, and the weight is less likely to go back on.

Home-cooking, meal planning and dietary monitoring may help

Dr Judy Kruger's mail study of those who had successfully lost weight and managed to keep it off, compared to those who lose weight but then regain it, had some similar results. The successful people were more active in everyday life and tended to take exercise for half an hour each day. They were less likely to use "over the counter" diet products and were more likely to plan meals, more likely to count calories or fat, measure food onto plates and to weigh themselves each day. In this sample, around a third were successful at keeping the weight off and those who did so were more likely to be in the age range 18-29 years. The least successful were aged 30-44 years. Men were more likely to keep weight off than women and those who had been at the top end of the weight scale had more difficulty maintaining their new weight.

You might think that spending more time in the kitchen cooking would not help keep weight off, but in fact "cooking or baking for fun" was done by 46% of those that kept the weight off and only 36% of those who regained weight. Although being in the kitchen means food is more accessible, it also means more home-made meals are being eaten. These will generally be more nutritious and healthier than fast food or restaurant meals. Home cooked food is less packed with calories than food bought away from home. A report on America's eating habits by Dr Elizabeth Frazao (US Dept of Agriculture) calculated that if food eaten away from home by Americans in 1995 had the same nutritional quality as home prepared food, then Americans would have each eaten 200 fewer calories per day. In addition, their calcium intake would have gone up by 7% and their fibre and iron intake would both have increased by 9%.

Reasons given for the failure to keep weight off included the increased cost of healthy food and difficulties finding healthy food to eat away from home, as well as being too busy or too tired to exercise.

Cutting down on frying food, drinking less diet soda and still eating some favourite foods can help prevent weight regain

Comparing women who lost weight and kept it off, with women who lost and then regained their weight, Susan Kaymen

(University of California) found that there were differences. Those who avoided weight regain made a decision to lose weight and then made a personal plan that fitted with their lifestyle. Some of these women used diet books and most ate more fruit and vegetables and foods that were low in fat and sugar. They avoided frying food and tried to still eat some of their favourite foods so that they did not feel deprived. Their approach to life problems tended to be "problem solving", in that they would confront problems and work to deal with them. Most of these women (90%) also took some form of regular exercise.

In contrast, the women who put weight back on were more likely to have lost the weight with the help of appetite suppressants or a very restrictive diet that was difficult to keep to. Diets that are difficult to keep to are probably going to be more difficult to maintain long term. Certainly, in medical treatment regimes, compliance is inversely related to the complexity of the regime. This implies that a straightforward diet of easily accessible food, might be preferable for weight maintenance.

These women who put the weight back on again saw "diet food" as special food and different to food that people normally eat. They cut out their favourite foods and they felt deprived as a consequence. They were more likely to miss breakfast and ate 5 snacks a day (compared to 1 or 2 for the weight maintainers) and more of them ate chocolate or sweets. Only a third of this group took regular exercise. The reasons given for the weight going back on included - having a negative life event that stopped them exercising or preparing food properly, or finding that they had gone back to their old ways without really noticing it and were surprised to find they had regained the weight. The way these women dealt with problems was different. They did not confront issues but reacted in a more emotional way, or with avoidance - such as wishing the situation would go away and eating or sleeping more. They had less friends or family to support them through troubles than those that managed to keep the weight off.

A control group, who had never had a weight problem, still thought about weight and said that they ate less or took more exercise if their clothes were getting tight. They drank fewer diet sodas (fizzy drinks) with only 8% drinking them, compared to 31% of those that had lost weight and managed to keep it off, or

41% of those who lost weight but then regained the weight.

These types of findings were similar to those found by Kristina Elfhag (University Hospital, Sweden) in a review of factors associated with weight loss maintenance. She found that the weight was more likely to stay off if there was healthy eating (to include breakfast and regular meals) an active lifestyle, and having lost more initial weight, including having reached a goal weight. These people also have more social support and are better at coping with stress than those who regain the weight. Putting the weight back on was associated with hunger, eating in response to stress and perhaps binge eating or dis-inhibited eating. It was also more likely if the person had previous weight cycling (weight going up and down frequently as diets are followed and then abandoned).

Dichotomous thinking & weight regain

Susan Bryne (Oxford University) interviewed women from community slimming clubs after they had lost 10% of their initial weight and then saw them every two months for a year. She found that the most powerful predictor of who would put the weight back on was "dichotomous thinking". This means tending to see all matters as "black and white" issues, with no shades of grey - not much evidence of a continuum. This pattern of thinking applied to all their thought processes and not just to issues related to food and diet. George Bush is often cited as an example of dichotomous thinking, "you're either with us or you're against us". Another example of dichotomous thinking would be "I'm either a success or a failure". It is an "all or nothing" way of looking at the world and all experiences tend to be divided into one of two opposing categories.

With regard to weight regain, you can see how thinking like this might not be helpful. The dichotomous thinker might think, "I've lost two stone but I'm still overweight. I'm never going to get to my goal weight. The diet is a total failure, so I might as well give up." Whereas someone who does not have this type of thinking might think, "I've lost two stone and I'm still not down to my goal weight but I'm looking and feeling a bit better so it is progress".

"I've eaten a cream cake. I'm never going to stick to my diet, it is not working - I'll give up" would be dichotomous thinking, as opposed to "I've eaten a cream cake. It's not good for the diet but it's not the end of the world. I'll take a bit of a walk this afternoon and have a healthy evening meal" which is more likely to give a positive result on weight maintenance, and makes abandonment of weight loss attempts less likely.

At the time that they had lost weight, those who were satisfied with the weight loss and felt that they had achieved their goal weight, then went on to be more likely to keep the weight off. Those who were not satisfied were more likely to put weight back on. Those who regained weight were more likely to have had weight fluctuation and were less vigilant with weight control.

Anecdotal comments recorded by Ms Byrne from the successful weight maintainers suggest that they adopted daily weighing and exercise as part of a new routine. They accepted that they had to watch the amount of fat, alcohol and fried food that they were consuming, because it was what they had to do to stay at the new weight. When faced with difficult life situations they coped without putting on weight.

In contrast, the people that put the weight back on made admissions such as being frightened to check their weight, because if they then found it had increased they would lose control and eat. They preferred not to know. They might have gone back to using the car and when confronted with stress, they ate to feel better. They tended to comfort eat, did not react immediately to any weight gain and were more likely to think of their own self-worth in terms of weight and shape. Of course, estimating your own value in terms of appearance is unhelpful and inaccurate. Losing four stone might make you slimmer and perhaps healthier but it will not make you cleverer, wittier, the life and soul of the party or lead to a wealthy, lavish lifestyle. Your family and friends will not love you more if you are slimmer (unless they are incredibly shallow). A sense of proportion when looking at weight issues is helpful.

Whereas having dichotomous thinking puts you at higher risk of weight gain, the second most powerful predictor of who would put on weight was the maximum lifetime weight. Those women with the higher maximum weight were more likely to regain the weight than those with lower maximum weight.

What sort of support works best in keeping weight off once it is lost?

To find whether "face to face" help with maintaining weight loss or internet chat groups are most helpful, 300 people who had lost around 20kg (44lbs) in the past two years were divided into 3 groups. The first was a control group that only received a quarterly newsletter with diet and exercise information. The second group received face to face help regularly in a hospital clinic, to help maintain their weight. The third group had group meetings in an internet chat room, these meetings led by the same staff who ran the hospital clinic.

The experiment, devised by Dr Rena Wing, also asked the volunteers to report weekly weight (apart from the control group). Those who had not put on any weight were given encouragement in the form of monthly "green gifts" such as green tea or a dollar bill. (I wonder if this would feel a bit patronising - maybe there is a cultural difference here between the US and the UK.) Those who had put on a small amount of weight were told to use problem solving skills to get their weight down. The volunteers who had put on over 2.3kg (5lbs) were told to restart weight loss attempts, either by using the method they had originally used, or by using a low fat diet and more activity. They were also encouraged to use a tool kit they were given at the start of the programme, containing aids such as a pedometer, a few cans of Slim Fast and books giving information on fat and calories.

The results were:

- Control group (Newsletter) - put on 4.9kg (11lbs) on average and 72% of them put on more than 2.3kg (5lbs).

- Face to face help - put on 2.5kg (5.5lbs) on average and only 46% of them put on more than 2.3kg (5lbs).

- Internet chat help - put on 4.7kg (10.4lbs) on average and 55% of them put on more than 2.3kg (5lbs).

So it seems from this, that people who lose weight stand a better chance of keeping it off with face to face help from an actual person, but use of the internet chat room will go some way to reducing the proportion who relapse.

Monitoring weight fairly frequently after it has been lost seems to help. Successful weight loss maintainers from Weight Watchers tend to start to take action to correct their weight when they are 3lbs (1.4kg) or less above their goal weight.

Self-help groups

Whether groups can help with weight loss maintenance depends on how well they are run. When they are well run and supportive they can be helpful - when they are poorly run there is the problem of "negative contagion". Listening to people who have failed to maintain or lose weight dwell on their failure, and listening at length to a description of the large amounts they have eaten, or small amounts of exercise that they have managed to take, could have a negative effect on other members of the group and discourage their own efforts. In the worst case, it could be competitive to see who has put on the most weight or over-indulged the most. A well run group would dwell more on the positive action that can be taken to correct a problem and provide encouragement and support, rather than a defeatist attitude. If a relapse occurs, looking at why it happened and what can be done to prevent it in future, as well as strategies to correct any weight gain, would be more helpful.

Summary - what is useful to know about weight loss maintenance?

Whilst everyone is an individual and what works for one person might not work for another, what data there is seems to indicate that there are some strategies which tend to be more successful at preventing weight regain than others. Walking seems to be helpful, as is eating food that is generally healthy, including food low in fat with plenty of vegetables, fruit, grains, pasta and cereals. Regular home prepared meals that include a breakfast (perhaps of cereal and fruit) eating some favourite foods and sticking to the same eating routine every day, with no variation at weekends, are good strategies. Avoiding frying food, drinking sodas, or eating chocolates and sweets, and being on full alert for the possibility of weight regain over the Christmas period, also seems worthwhile.

Getting some good quality support might help prevent weight regain, as might analysing how you think about food and diet. If you have a dichotomous approach you might want to try to be more flexible in this area. Trying not to value yourself in terms of shape and weight is helpful in maintaining weight loss. If you have a tendency to react emotionally to life problems, adopting a more problem solving approach might also help with weight control.

Regular weighing at least weekly, helps identify when a lapse has occurred, and tackling it at an early stage is preferable to waiting until a significant amount of weight has gone back on.

The last chapter in this book will deal with making a personal plan and I hope you will read to this chapter before making any major lifestyle decisions.

Chapter 6: The stigma of weight - who discriminates against larger people, and how do they cope with prejudice?

The stigma associated with excess weight is not talked about very much. However, there is a lot of evidence of prejudice against people of larger size, particularly affecting women at the upper end of the weight spectrum. The next chapter will help you to manage your own individual weight problem, but first it is useful have an idea of the prejudice that larger people face, the evidence that the discrimination is unfounded, and to look at strategies that people use to cope with the discrimination.

The advantage of being attractive

When I was training as a medical student, much of the teaching involved being sent off to various hospitals in order to experience the different specialties. This was usually done in groups of two, with another randomly selected student, for a couple of months at a time. The response of the permanent staff to finding they had students allocated to their ward varied from fairly helpful, through to indifferent - or making the students feel that they were in the way. However, when I was sent to study a few weeks of radiotherapy and ENT (ear, nose and throat) specialties, the quality of the teaching and helpfulness was astonishingly good. My co-student for these few weeks was female, tall, blonde, big eyes and by most male standards I suppose, very attractive. All the medical staff seemed exceptionally helpful.

Although I had, of course, realised that being attractive would perhaps make it more likely that you would be asked on dates, I had never considered that it could also enhance the quality of one's education. On one occasion we were queuing up to pay for lunch and a (male) doctor made a point of crossing the busy canteen to introduce himself and to offer to show us any interesting cases he came across. After he left, she looked at me and said "He was helpful, wasn't he?" I realised then that she lived in a totally different world to us ordinary looking people - one where people are particularly pleasant and helpful. She was also receiving a medical education that was superior to most of her fellow students. She seemed quite oblivious to this effect, so I didn't think it wise to enlighten her that her experiences probably were not representative of those of most students. It may be coincidence, but I believe that she finished the course one of a small handful of the 150 students who were considered to receive a distinction grade for her degree, so perhaps all that extra teaching helped.

There is quite a lot of evidence that more attractive people receive different treatment because of their looks. For instance, cadets at West Point military academy in the USA were rated for good looks (facial dominance) in the 1950's. Many years later, they were contacted to report their career history. There was found to be a "halo effect" of attractiveness, with the cadets' attractiveness ratings also predicting their military rank several years later. The better looking cadets were more likely to make the rank of General. (The exception was for men of below average performances, where the good looks appeared to be a handicap for promotion).

Attractive children also get judged more favourably than their less attractive friends. Karen Dion (University of Toronto) asked female students to rate the severity of misdemeanours committed by children aged 7, supplying the students with a photograph of either an attractive child or an unattractive child. Their judgements were more lenient if the child was attractive. When the child was unattractive, they thought it was more likely to indicate a long term tendency towards anti-social behaviour.

People tend to make positive assumptions about attractive people, seeing them as more able and with good social skills. If candidates for a job, for instance, are equally qualified, the attractive one is more likely to be hired than the unattractive candidate. If attractiveness affects people's reactions and they rate you more positively, what happens to those with an excess weight problem? Well, unfortunately, excess weight is generally viewed as unattractive and people tend to wrongly label the larger person with negative characteristics - such as stupid, ugly, mean, unhappy, lazy, socially isolated and lacking self-confidence. When college students were asked to rate photos of obese and non-obese women for attractiveness, with a score of 1 for unattractive, up to 9 for very attractive, the average score was 6.5 for the non-obese and 3.7 for the obese women.

Those of heavier weight have been described as "the last acceptable targets of discrimination and stigmatisation" and this seems to stem from the mistaken assumption that excess weight is a self-inflicted problem and the fault of the larger person.

The argument made by those supporting the prejudice, is that being overweight could adversely affect personality due to the larger person experiencing the unpleasant reactions of others to their weight. If attractive people live in a world where people tend to be kind and helpful and large people live in a world where people tend to judge them unkindly or are rude, could this, over time, affect the way their own personality develops into adulthood?

It has also been suggested that those who are extravert, emotionally stable and agreeable have "healthy" personality traits that protect them from life stresses that might lead to weight gain. Conscientiousness, in particular, could be related to healthy eating and exercise. The suggestion has been made that the prejudice is justified, if the less conscientious could, over time, gain weight. Is it possible that putting on extra weight could be a sign of being less conscientious?

The argument opposing this prejudice is the overwhelming medical evidence of a large genetic contribution to body weight and the fact that weight can be influenced by health problems.

Factors in the environment, such as food availability and social circumstances, also affect weight.

In a thorough piece of research, Prof. Mark Roehling (School of Labor and Industrial Relations, Michigan State University) undertook studies to find out whether there was any truth in the stereotypes that are often associated with being overweight. Is the larger person less conscientious, less agreeable, less stable and introverted, or are these stereotypes unfounded?

Prof. Roehling's study to decide this question was conducted on over 3,000 working age adults in the USA. It was particularly good in that it was not done on people who were a self-selected sample seeking treatment for weight loss (who can produce different results) but drew ordinary people from the general population.

The results were that there was no evidence that the overweight were any less agreeable or emotionally stable than the rest of the population. There was a small effect that found heavier men tended to be more agreeable than normal weight men, but this effect was so small as to be of no practical significance.

Similarly, there was a tiny effect with regard to the relationship between body size and conscientiousness and extraversion in women only (larger women found to be slightly less conscientious and less extravert). However, this was only large enough to explain less than 1% of the variance in extraversion and 1% of the variance in conscientiousness - effects too small to be of any practical significance. A second study, using more reliable and objective measures, failed to provide any evidence that overweight people score lower on either extraversion or conscientiousness.

The study concludes that body weight is not a practical predictor of personality traits such as conscientiousness and extraversion and it should not be used to predict personality in hiring situations.

Supporting this finding was work by Dr Beverly Brummett (Duke University Medical Centre), who tried to find out if personality could be related to the quality of diet eaten by married couples. There was no association between the quality of the diet and any of the personality traits such as neuroticism, extraversion, agreeableness and conscientiousness. The only correlation was that "openness" was associated with healthy eating habits. This is probably because those of more open personality are drawn more to novelty and variety in food, tending to lead to a more balanced diet.

It seems clear that there is no evidence to support discrimination against the larger person on personality grounds, yet there is widespread discrimination that has been compared to racism. In the case of the weight-challenged, this attitude seems to be more socially acceptable, more overt and more common.

Avoid conservative, racist men

At the heart of the prejudice against the larger person seems to be the false belief that being fat is the fault of the larger person - it is somehow due to lack of willpower or a personality defect. Although there is much evidence that none of this is true, the general public does not seem to be aware of this, and the stigma of excess weight continues.

Those who believe in the "Protestant work ethic", that hard work leads to success and poor effort to failure, may see larger people as failing to control their weight and think that they deserve to be stigmatised. Perhaps some people may be critical of weight because they want to maintain power over others and increase their own status in the process. Alternatively, they might mistakenly think that their criticism will be helpful, and will encourage the larger person to make more effort to lose weight. Some people are afraid of becoming large themselves and meeting a larger person reminds them of their fears. It has been found that those who are more concerned with the possibility of gaining weight themselves, are more likely to be prejudiced against overweight women.

Over 1,000 students were surveyed about their attitude to larger people in the USA by Christian Crandall. He found that those with the strongest anti-fat attitudes tended to be politically and ideologically conservative, racist, in favour of capital punishment and they did not approve of non-traditional marriage. These findings were stronger among men than women. Those with anti-fat attitudes were also more likely to be authoritarian and less accepting of other's behaviour. Interestingly, the person's anti-fat attitudes were unrelated to their own weight situation - although if an overweight conservative woman had anti-fat attitudes, she was also more likely to suffer from low self-esteem. It is surprising that anti-fat attitudes are found not just among the normal weight population, but equally among larger people. For instance, a small study sent students to see landlords about accommodation in the USA. All offered to rent to the normal weight students but just over half would rent to the obese students. The weight of the landlord did not seem to be related to the likelihood of this discriminatory behaviour.

Part of the problem with discrimination against the larger person is that to some extent people are not aware that they are doing it - it has become an acceptable attitude. Once people are aware of these stereotypes, they can then consciously override their tendency to prejudice. Awareness of prejudice is the first step to reducing prejudice.

Here, I must confess that before I started researching this book, although I am certainly not a racist conservative in favour of capital punishment, I probably was guilty of believing some of the general myths about weight. I wasn't fully aware of the evidence on genetic and environmental causes of the problem, and was under the impression that those who had a weight problem were just eating the wrong foods or maybe had other difficulties causing them to eat more. I have to say, that having extensively researched the subject, my attitudes have changed considerably.

What sort of discrimination occurs?

Larger people are discriminated against in shops, education, employment, transport and in the media, and the greater the weight problem, the greater the likelihood of experiencing discrimination. Women suffer much more from weight-based discrimination than men, and at relatively lower levels of excess weight. Society adversely judges women for their excess weight to a much greater extent than it judges men. (Men tend to be discriminated against if they are of short stature, as opposed to heavier, but this is not within the remit of this book.)

Rebecca Puhl and Kelly Brownell (Yale University) have done much of the work examining the stigma that goes with being overweight or obese. They have found that the most common problems encountered include the low expectations other people have of people of larger size, unpleasant comments from children, seat belts too small, unpleasant comments by family and others, causing embarrassment to their family, being avoided, stared at, or workplace discrimination. Nine per cent say they have been attacked because of their weight.

Who are the people most commonly found to be guilty of insulting behaviour towards larger people? Family members, doctors, classmates, sales assistants and friends are the most common sources of insult, followed by work colleagues, parents, restaurant staff and employers. Less common sources of insult are siblings, teachers, police, sons and daughters and mental health professionals. It is a fairly wide-ranging list.

Rebecca Puhl also asked about the worst experiences that overweight or obese people had with stigmatisation. She found that these were with close relationships such as friends, parents or spouses - for instance, being called unpleasant names or being insulted. Most of the people she questioned wished that the rest of the population would realise that they were not lazy, that obesity has multiple causes and losing weight is very difficult. They also would like people to know about physical difficulties, such as not being able to fit into public transport seating, and that being stigmatised and insulted could make them feel depressed or hurt. Larger people don't want to be judged for their appearance and would like people to be more supportive, and to have an increased proportion of larger people on television and in the media.

Shopping - should you carry a diet coke?

Years ago, when I was a student, I had a holiday job in a coffee shop. One of the duties was to make milkshakes for customers. This involved mixing milk, fruit syrup and a scoop of ice-cream in a jug and then putting it under a frothing machine before pouring it into a tall glass. I'm now ashamed to admit it, but when a large person would ask for a milkshake, I would put a very small scoop of ice cream into the mix. If it was an average weight person, I would be a lot more generous. Yet they were all paying the same, and in retrospect the customer was entitled to have the same shake as everyone else. My excuse for the ice cream related discrimination is that at the time I did not realise that obesity was largely due to factors beyond personal control and I thought I was being helpful.

Eden King (Rice University) did a series of tests to see how shop assistants treated their larger customers in a shopping mall in Houston, Texas. She used a group of women who were of average weight and height. She selected them for their round faces, so that they would look convincing in a "fat suit" of size 22 (UK size 24). The women went into shops, sometimes wearing the fat suit and sometimes without. On some occasions they were dressed in casual clothes (including a sweatshirt), and on others they were wearing smart professional clothes (with a jacket). They had instructions to browse for a few minutes and if no assistant approached them to find one, and ask for a couple of recommendations for a gift for their sister's birthday. After receiving the advice they thanked the assistant, said they needed more time to decide and left the store.

It was found that for all sizes and clothing styles, the customer was greeted and given recommendations, but that there was a greater level of covert interpersonal discrimination towards the larger customer. There was less smiling, less friendliness, more rudeness and a greater likelihood of prematurely ending the conversation. Wearing the professional smart clothes reduced the amount of discrimination, compared to wearing the casual clothes.

They went on to do a further study, just using the casual clothes, with and without the fat suit but with other differences. In one scenario, the customer would be drinking a high calorie ice cream drink whilst asking for advice. As part of the conversation, they would mention how good the drink was, that they were not on a diet and how they could never consider doing a half marathon. In the second scenario, the drink would be replaced by a diet coke, and included in the conversation was the fact that the coke tasted good, they were on a diet and had just done a half marathon.

The findings were that the customer with the diet coke received better treatment. The assistant smiled more, was friendlier and less likely to prematurely end the conversation.

Perhaps the assistant felt the customer with the high calorie drink was seen to be providing high justification for discrimination towards them, whereas the assistant felt less justified in being unfriendly towards the customer with the diet coke.

A final study approached real shoppers as they came out of stores. They were asked to fill in an anonymous short survey about their shopping experience. At the same time, the researcher covertly evaluated their body size. The larger shoppers also reported more interpersonal discrimination, in that they experienced less smiling, less eye contact, more rudeness and they found that staff were more likely to prematurely end conversations. They spent less money than they had intended to, and there was a slight tendency to spend less time in the store. They also said that they would be less likely to return to the store in the future. With the increasing proportion of larger people in our society, the retail trade might want to take steps to remedy this situation. As well as being morally right, it would help them to make more profit.

Although it would be great if weight based discrimination were ended, in the meantime larger people wanting to improve their level of service might consider dressing smartly and giving the impression they are dieting, which makes people feel less justified in being rude. Carrying a diet drink around is, to my mind, a step too far.

Education - larger pupils may do less well

In the USA, if you are obese you are less likely to be accepted into college than an average weight person, particularly if you are a woman. As well as having this disadvantage, you are less likely to get financial support from your parents, especially if you are female. Research (by Crandall), found that larger female students are more likely to have to get their financial support from sources such as savings or jobs, whilst average weight students rely mainly on their family for money. Daughters of politically conservative parents suffer the strongest anti-fat bias and are least likely to get financial help.

It seems unlikely that parents are looking at their offspring and consciously deciding that they will pay for the education of their normal weight children, be slightly less generous to the overweight sons and be mean to their larger daughters. It is possible that the adverse treatment is due to a subconscious desire to punish their daughters for "failing to control their appetite". The daughters may be subject to the anti-fat attitudes that go with the belief that the overweight are to blame for their problem.

Dr Nina Karnehed looked at the education record of over 700,000 Swedish men born between 1952 and 1973. She found that obese men do worse in the education system than average weight men, even when adjustments were made for intelligence, parents' education and socioeconomic group. At school, at the age of 18, the larger men were awarded lower marks than would have been expected from their intelligence tests, less of them went on to university and fewer graduated than average weight men. These results may be the result of discrimination - possibly because the teachers have lower expectations of their larger pupils and encourage them less?

Getting a place in graduate school in the USA could depend on your size. Seventy public health administrators were sent identical curricula vitae and covering letters asking about the student's chances of getting into graduate school and finding subsequent employment. Some received a photo of an obese woman with the letter, some a normal weight woman and some no photo at all. Those that got the letter with the photo of the larger woman were less likely to reply than those who received the normal weight photo or no photo. The chances of getting into college and finding subsequent work, were described as significantly reduced, when the larger weight photo was sent.

Sometimes the discrimination is much more overt. Sharon Russell was expelled from her nursing course in the USA in 1985, because she was a large woman and she had failed to lose weight. She had performed well academically and was one year from graduating, but was subject to harassment about her weight from staff and students. She went on to get her degree from another college. The Supreme Court awarded her financial damages for wrongful dismissal, intentional infliction of emotional distress and discrimination.

Employment

Hiring – depends who you sit next to

Research using professional personnel consultants and students has found that attractive candidates are preferred to equally qualified but unattractive candidates. The attractive people are viewed as more likeable and more likely to be intelligent and to have greater skills.

As excess weight is generally considered unattractive and attractive people are hired preferentially, the larger person is at a disadvantage when it comes to finding a job. This disadvantage seems to be greater the larger the weight problem and affects women much more than men.

This is borne out by findings of the National Association to Advance Fat Acceptance (NAAFA). They found that those members who were only about 33% above the standard weight for their size did not have much of a problem, but those who were double the desirable weight for their size reported more discrimination. They were more likely to have been advised to lose weight by colleagues or bosses and some were only employed conditional upon them losing weight. It was this larger group who were more likely to try and hide their weight by applying for jobs over the phone, rather than in person. They also felt that they had less self-confidence - these effects were much more marked in women than men. Other studies found that around half of obese women have been targeted by derogatory humour or unpleasant remarks at work and they felt that they had been refused employment, missed out on promotion or been sacked/fired because of their size.

Just sitting next to a woman with a weight problem can reduce your chances of getting a job - such is the level of discrimination against the larger person. Dr Michelle Hebl (Rice University) devised a study which took place in an airport lounge in Houston, which had these surprising results. Researchers approached equal numbers of male and female professionally dressed middle-aged travellers, who were waiting for a mid-week flight in business hours. They were asked to look at a man's job application and curriculum vitae and judge if he was suitable for hiring. Included in the application was a picture of the man, supposedly at a social function hosted by the company. In one of the photos he was sitting next to a size 8 (UK size 12) woman in business clothes. In another photo he was sitting next to the same woman, also professionally dressed, but the difference was that she was wearing a fat suit and appeared to be a size 22 (UK size 24). The travellers were not told whether they were strangers or whether there was any relationship. The results were striking. The man was rated lower in professional qualities and interpersonal skills by those that had seen the photo of him with the larger woman (compared to those who had seen him with the average sized woman). They also rated him as less suitable for hiring.

In a further study, a series of volunteers would sit in a waiting room, having been told he/she was taking part in research about hiring decisions. A man was sitting opposite, playing the role of another "volunteer", who was later chosen to be evaluated for his hiring qualities. Sometimes he would be alone - on other occasions a woman of average weight would come and sit next to him and on yet other occasions the same woman wearing a fat suit would sit next to him. In some cases they gave the impression they were strangers and in others that they were girlfriend and boyfriend. Again, the results were surprising, with the volunteers rating the man less suitable for hiring when he had been sitting next to the larger woman compared to the average weight woman or when he was alone. They thought he was less professional and had less interpersonal skills.

These experiments seem to show that just sitting next to a large woman can cause other people to judge you adversely. This kind of "stigma by association" has been described in other areas, such as against gay people, where those who associate with the stigmatised person face negative interpersonal and professional outcomes. However, there is something of a difference here, in that the stigma occurred whether they were thought to be friends or strangers - implying that the stigma associated with excess weight is of some significance.

Similar results were found by Regina Pingitore (Chicago Medical School) when students were shown videotapes of actors undergoing employment interviews, with and without the addition of fat suits that added just two stone in appearance. Using the suit showed that the applicant's body weight was responsible for around 35% of the variance in hiring decisions, with the bias more noticeable for heavier women than men. Other studies have shown that being overweight would go against the hiring of a PE teacher in the public schools of the USA, no matter how well qualified they were.

Women are 16 times more likely to report weight discrimination at work than men and very large people in professional jobs are more likely to be discriminated against than those in non-professional jobs.

There seems to be little doubt that a person with a significant weight problem is at a disadvantage at the hiring stage, especially if they are female. This disadvantage gets greater with the extent of the weight problem and is more apparent in professional jobs.

Wages - you earn less if you are big, especially if you are female - unless you live in Australia

In the USA, plain people earn less than average looking people, who earn less than good-looking people. The wage difference is 10% more for being attractive than plain.

English society seems to find it acceptable for a man to be overweight. Overweight men get the highest wages, but a woman will have a lower wage if she is overweight. A survey in England in 2006 showed that women earn most if they are a normal weight, 2% less if they are underweight and 12% less if they are morbidly obese. (Excess weight is categorised as overweight, then obese, then morbidly obese at the most extreme.) For English men, the highest wages go to the overweight, and the lowest to those in the underweight and morbidly obese categories.

Prof. James Sargent looked at the relationship between obesity and height in adolescence and subsequent earnings at the age of 23, in British people. Those women who are obese at the age of 16 earn less than normal weight women at the age of 23 years, even if they have become normal weight themselves by that time. He suggests that events that happen around the age of 16 might be causing this long lasting effect. There was no weight related loss of earnings in men, although they do earn more if they are tall. What happens to a girl around the age of 16 that might reduce her future income due to her size? Perhaps larger girls tend to be directed towards employment that pays less, or receive less encouragement to pursue a career? Unfortunately, this study did not look at the reasons for the loss of income.

Similar findings were reported in the USA in the 1990's, with women who were overweight or obese between the ages of 16 and 25, having a family income of almost $7,000 dollars a year less than normal weight women. Here, the difference was mostly because they were 20% less likely to get married than a normal weight woman. If they did get married, their husband's income was likely to be lower. The size of American men did not have so much effect on their wages.

So the general picture seems to be that larger women tend to get paid less. There is much less of an effect for larger men - where overweight can be associated with higher pay (as long as it does not become obesity). In the USA, overweight men are over-represented amongst top company Chief Executive Officers, but obese men are under-represented (although among lawyers the overweight ones are paid less than the normal weight lawyers). The wage penalty is much greater at the extreme weights such as morbid obesity, compared to mild obesity. In general, the loss of wages for size is more of a problem towards the top of the career ladder, with more discrimination in managerial and professional jobs.

There is some variation in the wage cut associated with weight, depending where you live. In Finland, obese women in white collar positions earn nearly a third less than their colleagues, and there is no cut in income at all for men, regardless of their body weight. However, self-employed obese Finnish women buck the general trend. For these women, the greater the body size, the greater the income. Dr Siro Sarlio-lahteenkorva (University of Helsinki) who conducted this study suggested that larger Finnish women might be better off self-employed, because they are then not subject to employer discrimination.

The best place to work, if you have a weight problem, might be Australia, where a survey in 2009 showed that there was no wage penalty for being overweight or obese in the Australian labour market, regardless of gender. Maybe Australians do not discriminate in the way that other nations do? 36% of Australians are overweight and 22% are obese, making up over half the workforce. Either attitudes in Australia are changing, or there might be a cultural difference between Australians and those living in the USA and Europe? The same study showed that there was no effect between height and wages in women, but in men, an extra 5cm in height was worth $950 a year.

Can weight affect promotion and career prospects?

The evidence is that weight does have an effect on career, but generally this is a problem that affects women more than men. Larger women are less likely to be promoted and are treated more harshly in disciplinary situations.

Human Resource Professionals in the UK were surveyed in 2005. Nearly half thought that being obese had an adverse effect on employee output and a third thought that obesity was a valid medical reason to refuse to employ someone. An astonishing 11% thought that they could sack/fire someone just for being obese, 15% said that they would be less likely to promote someone who was obese, and 12% said that obese people would not be suitable for jobs where they would meet customers.

When over 100 managers and supervisors were asked to rate hypothetical employees for promotion (by Dr James Bordieri), the employees who were obese or suffering from depression were rated lower than an average employee who was normal weight and not disabled. However, employees who had cancer, an amputation, diabetes, poor vision or facial burns were rated similarly to normal weight non-disabled employees. Presumably the discrimination occurred against the heavier employees and the depressed because the managers felt they were to blame for their condition.

Obese sales professionals tend to get allocated the less favourable selling territories, although not in telesales where there is less personal client interaction. A study by Professor J Bellizi (Arizona State University) showed that in disciplinary situations, an overweight sales woman will be dealt with more harshly than her normal weight colleagues. However, there is no difference for men - in disciplinary situations their weight is irrelevant.

Women in the British Civil Service are also disadvantaged by weight. Over a period of several years, 14% of obese female staff were promoted, compared to nearly 22% of the non-obese women. There is no discrimination in promotion for obese men.

Being large can also lead to loss of a job. In one self-reported survey in the USA among obese people, 17% reported being sacked or pressured into resigning because of their weight.

These statistics highlight the level of prejudice against the larger person, particularly against women. As we have already discussed, there is no objective evidence that larger people are in any way less agreeable, or less conscientious, than other employees. So this leads us to our next question -

How do employers justify discriminating against their larger employees?

Various reasons have been given by employers for weight-related discrimination. They are generally offensive reasons, but in order to combat prejudice it is probably necessary to confront the opinions, so you might forgive my reproducing them here.

Employers were found to consider that overweight job applicants and employees were lazy, less able to get along with colleagues, less competent than average weight people, lack self-discipline and are more likely to be absent, have emotional problems and poor hygiene, in a review undertaken by Prof Mark Roehling (Michigan State University).

Other employers have given the excuse that although they do not have any adverse views on larger persons themselves, they have to discriminate against them because they are under pressure from others to do so. (This is a poor argument - a bit like saying, "I'm not racist or sexist, but my boss is, so I have to embrace the prejudice.") The increased cost of health care in the USA (though not in the UK where employers do not pay for health care) is sometimes cited as a reason for not wishing to employ larger people, or that customers will buy less from staff involved in sales if the staff are large and the customers have anti-fat attitudes themselves.

Is there any truth in these prejudices? It seems that there is very little. As we have already discussed, research has disproved the notion that larger people have a less agreeable or conscientious personality than normal weight people. One study of employees selling life insurance even found that heavier employees were better and had higher sales, than the normal weight employees.

So the claims that larger people are less conscientious, lazy, less competent, lack self-discipline or have emotional difficulties have been dismissed as wrong by research in this area. What about sick leave? Excess weight has been associated with an increase in health problems, but are employers justified in saying that larger people will spend too much time off sick and should be discriminated against because of this?

The evidence on sick leave is mixed, for instance:

- In Kentucky, a study of manufacturing companies found there was just over 1% loss of productivity in those who were at the extreme end of the heavy weight spectrum, as they took longer to do physically demanding tasks. However, overweight employees took less time off sick than all other employees, including normal weight employees.

- In Belgium, a study of over 20,000 workers found that there was only an increase in sick leave in the very highest categories of weight excess.

- A 10 year study of over 4,000 employees of the Shell petrochemical company found that normal weight employees took 2.6 days sick each year, the overweight 4.2 days and the obese 7.2 days.

- Whitehall (London) civil servants who are obese take 25% more short term sick leave (less than 7 days) and 60% more long term sick leave. However, this was a study of public sector office workers in London and may not translate to other sectors.

- A recent study of over 10,000 people in the USA (of various professions and worksites) found the normal weight person visited the doctor 3.05 times each year and took 4 days off sick - compared to 3.93 doctor visits and 6 days off sick for the obese person.

- A review of sick leave studies was done by Kristian Neovius (Karolinska Institutet) who found that there is no convincing evidence that workers who are overweight take more time off sick than normal weight workers. Once the weight reaches the level that could be described as obese, workers take 1-3 extra days compared to normal weight workers in the US, and in Europe they take an extra 10 days.

The picture is further complicated by the fact that in the USA sick leave is often unpaid, whereas in Europe it is more likely to be paid for by the employer. It gives more incentive for the American worker to go into work when they are sick and Americans take around one fifth of the sick leave taken by European workers. It seems that other factors apart from weight are likely to influence sick leave much more strongly, including the country involved, whether sick leave is paid or unpaid and the culture of the working environment, including whether it is public or private sector. Public sector workers in the UK take more sick leave than private sector workers.

There is not much of a case for discriminating against the merely overweight as the evidence for excess sick leave is poor and some studies have even suggested that being overweight is associated with taking reduced sick leave. At the extreme end of the obesity scale there does seem to be a slight statistical possibility of extra sick leave. However, when faced with an individual employee, the notion that they might take a couple of extra days leave each year is of little significance, compared to their general suitability for a job. You might as well, for instance, ask prospective employees whether they go skiing or rock climbing (both sports which have a risk of injury and a possible need for sick leave) and then exclude these people. This is not a course of action which most would consider reasonable.

What about the employer's concerns that if they employ larger staff in sales, their sales will go down if customers are prejudiced against the overweight? There is some experimental evidence that customers may initially react in this way. Students were asked to rate a store experimentally - when the salesperson was presented as obese, the store was described as having a poorer image and as being less successful. However, these experiments, where people have limited information, lead them to rely on stereotypes to form an opinion. In a real life situation, any initial adverse impression of the salesperson would be likely to be quickly overturned if the salesperson was helpful and good at their job. Most customers would prefer a good, well informed, salesperson who happened to be large, than a slender salesperson who was unhelpful and knew nothing about the product.

Is there ever any justification for choosing staff on the basis of size? It seems there are a few occasions - for instance, when various sized models were used to advertise a diet drink, the thinner models were associated with a more positive brand image and increased intention to buy the drink. However, when the drink was not a diet drink there was no relationship between the model size and brand image or intention to buy the drink. The instances where discrimination by size by employers is justified, is limited to very few - such as to advertise diet drinks.

Is it legal to discriminate against the larger employee?

Catherine McDermott was refused employment by Xerox Corporation as a systems analyst because she was obese. She was 5ft 6" tall and 249lbs (17 stone/113kg) and although she was healthy, they would not employ her because she might develop problems with her health in the future. The case went to court and the court ordered Xerox to hire Ms McDermott, compensate her for lost income and pay $1,000 for hurt, humiliation and mental anguish, having ruled that her obesity was actually a disability under New York law. Unfortunately, the legal proceedings took 11 years, by which time she was 67 years old and no longer wanted the job.

Joe Gimello was a manager of a rent-a-car firm in the USA. He had a family history of obesity and he had always had an excess weight problem. He started work at the weight of 225lbs (16 stone/102kg) and over the next 4 years his work was described as outstanding and he was promoted. A new regional manager was then appointed who said he "wasn't promotable" because of his size and weight. He thought that if Joe was promoted he would, "hire fat sloppy people". He directed remarks at him such as to enquire whether he was "still eating the doughnuts?" Joe was sacked from his job at a weight of approximately 23 stone (324lbs/147kg) after 5 years of employment and he took the case to court. He was ordered to be paid back pay, $10,000 for pain, humiliation and suffering and nearly $3,000 for incidental compensatory damages, as well as his legal fees.

There are many similar cases documented, mostly in the USA, often involving airlines that have sacked/fired female flight attendants for putting on small amounts of weight. In the USA, claims against employers seem to be won either by claiming that obesity is a disability, or in the case of women, by claiming discrimination. Some think that morbid obesity (the heaviest weight category) could be considered a disability as it severely limits life activities, but the counter-argument in court tends to be that obesity is voluntary and the position varies from state to state.

In the UK, there are no "anti-fat" discrimination laws but it is illegal to sack people just because of their size. The employer would have to prove that it had a negative effect on business. If the excess weight is due to an underlying medical condition the employee could be covered by the Disability Discrimination Act.

"When aliens come they will eat the fat ones first"

A law that soon became known as the "purple hair law" or the "ugly ordinance" that prohibited the discrimination against people on the basis of appearance (including height, weight, physical characteristics, age, gender, race, disability or religion) was proposed in 1992 by Santa Cruz City Council, California. The thinking behind the law was that people should not be judged on the basis of stereotypes. They should be judged on the basis of their ability to do the job, in the case of employment, or to pay rent in the case of accommodation. At first, the response of the population was one of worry about the possible consequences of such a law. "If someone had 14 earrings in their ears and their nose - and who knows where else - and spiky green hair and smells like a skunk, I don't know why I have to employ them," said restaurant owner, Kathy Manoff. The law was modified to forbid discrimination on the basis of physical characteristics that are not under personal control and this includes weight. It is, however, still legal to discriminate against those who have tattoos, nose piercing or unsuitable clothes.

After a billboard was placed around San Francisco City advertising a fitness company, with the slogan, "When Aliens Come They Will Eat The Fat Ones First", it caused such offence that a similar law was passed in San Francisco prohibiting weight discrimination. An exception was made for jobs that have a physical requirement, such as fire-fighting.

Discrimination on grounds of weight is probably best combated with this type of legislation. The alternative legal route of trying to classify excess weight as a disability and then using disability discrimination legislation is much less preferable. Larger people do not consider themselves to be disabled and it could lead to further stigmatisation of those with excess weight. The thought, for instance, of labelling obese children as disabled due to their weight, is quite unkind.

In my opinion, discrimination should be outlawed for physical characteristics beyond a person's control and this should include weight.

The Professor of Economics at Harvard, Robert Barro, takes the opposite view and argues that it is a good thing to discriminate on grounds of appearance - employers should be able to choose on looks, just as much as they might choose on characteristics such as intelligence. He feels that appearance is a legitimate job qualification, particularly on television and in films. He thinks flight attendants should be selected on appearance, as it is valued by customers but he appears to think that all flight attendants are women, and all customers are heterosexual men.

As he is unlikely to be applying for a job as a flight attendant, he might not be too concerned by discrimination in favour of the attractive. However, what if it were a requirement that Professors of Economics should be particularly attractive, in order to hold the attention of their students during lectures? I doubt he would be quite so keen to discriminate in favour of the beautiful then.

He would, no doubt, point out that a good understanding of economics was far more important to the role than looks - just as a flight attendant is employed to have skills in customer care, serving food and drinks, checking tickets, dealing with medical and airborne emergencies and more recently, responding to possible terrorist threats. Looking pretty or thin is certainly not on my list of requirements for a flight attendant.

He also supported the settlement of the case of "Hooters", when it was allowed to continue to restrict its serving staff to attractive young women. This is an American restaurant chain that employs attractive young women who must wear a uniform of shorts and tight fitting tops. The tops have a picture of an owl and the word "hooters" across the chest. The two o's of the word hooters appear over the breast regions. The waitresses are required to smile and the chain's motto is "Hooter's - More Than A Mouthful". I suppose one could feel sorry for a man that needed his flight attendants to be attractive and his waitresses to serve food wearing clothes that are sexually suggestive. He doesn't say whether he would be keen to wear such a uniform suggesting sexual availability himself, or whether he would be happy for his wife or daughter to be judged by appearances when applying for a job.

In a civilised society, there is a good case for legislation that prohibits discrimination on the basis of physical characteristics that are not within a person's control - and that includes weight. The criteria for selecting an employee should always be whether they are the most competent person for the job and have the necessary skills - not do I, personally, like the look of them.

What can the larger person do to counteract the stigma associated with their size in an employment situation?

Being well qualified for the job can help overcome the stigma associated with weight. When clients asking for counselling from a university service were offered a choice of poorly qualified counsellors from a brochure of normal weight and overweight staff, the clients saw the normal weight counsellor as more expert and trustworthy. When all the counsellors were presented as highly qualified, the ratings were the same regardless of weight.

Another study showed that in a lab situation, a qualified overweight person was preferred to a normal weight unqualified person, but in this instance when the qualifications were equal the larger candidate was rated as less suitable. It seems in these sorts of experimental situations, people probably rely more on stereotypes because of the lack of other real life input.

The research suggests that in an employment situation the poor view sometimes associated with excess weight can be overcome by presenting good qualifications and a history of achievement. Until attitudes change, the person with a weight problem might wish to obtain extra qualifications or skills and to focus on appearing competent. They might also consider whether there is any benefit in mentioning on job applications or at interviews some evidence of fitness, if the appropriate situation arises. Giving an impression of sporting hobbies or gym membership might help dispel some of the stereotypical ideas associated with larger people.

Do not mention a weight problem at interview though. Some research in this area by Prof Roehling suggests that larger candidates who do not mention their weight are viewed more favourably than those that do mention their condition. This is in contrast to those with a physical disability, who are viewed more favourably when they do mention the condition.

The best advice to a larger person at interview might be to wear professional clothes and to avoid referring to a weight problem. If appropriate, drop into the conversation some reference to participating in sport or exercise, and try to present yourself as well qualified and competent.

Media - overwhelmingly prejudiced

Can you think of an overweight leading character at the movies? It is not easy and I cannot think of any leading roles for larger women in films. Among male characters, I could only come up with the late John Candy. Larger characters are often featured eating, and around food. For instance, John makes pancakes in *Uncle Buck*. Other characters might complain about their weight whilst actually being a healthy normal weight. In the *Bridget Jones* movie, Bridget tells her diary she is 136lbs (9 stone

10lbs/62kg) and "obviously will lose 20lbs (9kg)". The actor playing her appears to be about 5ft 4" tall, which according to weight charts means that her maximum healthy weight is 10 stone 7lbs (67kg), so she is well within the normal healthy weight for her height and is not overweight at all.

On television, the larger women that come to mind tend to be either comediennes, such as Dawn French, or cooks. *Two Fat Ladies,* was the title of one UK cookery series, featuring two larger cooks. Larger women seem almost exclusively confined to comedy and cookery in the UK.

Dr Bradley Greenberg (Michigan State University) studied nearly 300 episodes of 10 fictional series, shown at prime viewing time in the USA. He found that larger people are under-represented, with the proportion of larger people on television less than half that found in the population as a whole. Larger characters are found more often in comedies than dramas, and tend to be the target of humorous remarks. They are more likely to be older, members of ethnic minorities, unemployed or unmarried, and are more likely to be shown eating. They are less likely to be shown in a romantic or leadership role.

In an analysis of 18 situation comedies by Prof. Gregory Fouts (University of Calgary), underweight women were over-represented and very few were above average weight. The higher the weight of a female character, the more unpleasant remarks will be directed towards her by the male characters and audiences laugh at this. However, female characters are no more likely to make a negative comment about a male character if he is heavier. This reinforces the message that it is fine for men to be critical of a woman's weight, and larger women should expect to be harassed in this manner.

Susan Himes (University of S. Florida) analysed 25 movies including *Love Actually, Mean Girls, Shrek* and *Dodgeball* and ten TV series, including *Will and Grace, Friends* and *The Golden Girls*. Male characters were 3 times more likely to issue negative verbal remarks or indulge in anti-fat humour targeted towards larger characters, than were female characters.

In the UK, a similar gender difference seems to be happening on our television, with female presenters and newsreaders in particular, often appearing painfully thin. This does not seem to happen with the male presenters, who are still permitted on our screens when plump, middle-aged, grey and wrinkled. Why are women not allowed the same freedom to age, or to put on weight? I suspect it is because network bosses are still predominately middle-aged men in suits, who on some level feel it is acceptable for men to put on weight and get old (like themselves) but women should be young, pretty, thin and non-threatening. Probably this attitude is partly rooted in chauvinism. Newsreaders are employed to read the news or for their presenting skills - if they are good at their job, what can it matter if they are overweight? One explanation that has been suggested is that as women have moved into jobs that were traditionally done by men, they have had to emulate their "straight up and down" physique and eliminate their natural curves. Of course, these stick thin people are poor role models for growing teenage girls and young women, as it gives the message that if you want to be successful and on television, you have to be underweight.

Even worse, is the current fashion for reality shows on television. Larger people are subjected to a punishing regime of diet and exercise in an effort to lose weight, for public entertainment. Most of these shows perpetuate the myth that the larger person is at fault as a result of a character flaw, despite the overwhelming evidence that this is not the case. In the UK, one of these shows is called *Fat Families*. In just the first part of one of these programmes, the presenter said that he wanted to turn 4 singers "from blobs to bodies" and described them as "a colossal quartet, fatty foursome and flabby friends with backstage passes to porky-ville". He then tried to upset them by presenting them with disgusting food, such as chicken heads and sheep's eyeballs, telling them that they needed to take responsibility for what they were eating.

Further humiliation followed with a close-up camera shot of their bodies wearing only underwear, in front of a mirror. He then takes them to a clinic, where they are reduced to tears by being told they are at risk of strokes and heart attacks and so forth. Later he revisits them, "lardy ladies, naughty girls, to see what they've been shovelling down their cake-holes". They are made to sit in a school room and eat food with doll's cutlery to slow their eating, followed by a street dancing class for exercise, where they dance far better than the presenter. The last follow up meeting is only 8 weeks after the first visit, and each has lost around 2 stone (28lbs/13kg) in weight. They are then given a makeover, and told they are now "sassy singing sensations".

This type of disrespectful and frankly rude attitude to people with a weight problem could be damaging to the participants who have to endure public humiliation. It gives the message very clearly, to the general public, that it is permissible to be downright rude about someone's weight.

Children's media also has a problem with size. In one study of the top 25 movies for children, around two-thirds associated larger size with traits such as being unfriendly, evil or unattractive. *Cinderella* and *The Little Mermaid* had the most negative messages about size.

Children's books give less emphasis to body size than films but it still does occur. In the *Harry Potter* books, the evil family with which Harry lives have a father described as "a big, beefy man with hardly any neck". The bullying son (Dudley) has "blond hair (which) lay smoothly on his thick, fat head". "Harry often said he looked like a pig in a wig". His walk is described as "waddling". Perhaps J K Rowling realised that she was stigmatising the character and the film actor, because in the later books, Dudley's weight becomes attributed more to muscle bulk than fat.

Transport - a minefield of public humiliation?

Arthur Berkowitz had to stand for the whole of a seven hour flight from Anchorage to Philadelphia, when the large passenger sitting next to him made it impossible for him to sit down. Both arm rests had to be raised so that he could sit down and his body also filled half of Mr Berkowitz's seat. The passenger apologised profusely to Mr Berkowitz but he was undoubtedly humiliated and Mr Berkowitz was severely inconvenienced. This is not an isolated incident of size being a problem on planes. The actor and director, Kevin Smith, was removed from a Southwest Airline flight from Oakland to Burbank, California. He was told that he did not fit into a single seat, even though he could put both arm rests down. He vowed never to fly with this airline again.

The attitude of airlines both to the size of their staff and their passengers seems to be, on the whole, extremely poor. With half the people in the USA overweight, the airlines seem slow to appreciate that if they do not increase the size of their seating and change their corporate attitude to size, they risk alienating a large proportion of the paying public.

Many airlines now force passengers to buy an additional seat if they cannot sit in the seat with the arm rests down, and secure the seat belt with only a single extender. Sometimes the cost of the extra seat is refunded if the plane takes off with empty seats. Until the attitude to larger customers changes, all the weight-challenged person can do is to contact the airline prior to booking, to find out the airline's policy. Sometimes they are advised to avoid peak travel times and travel when there are more likely to be spare seats, or to upgrade to business class where the seats are larger.

The Dennys restaurant chain was sued by Gary Sellick after they failed to provide him with a wide enough or armless chair. They caused him emotional distress due to the public humiliation he felt over his treatment by the waitress. He claimed $100,000 compensation plus $1.2 million in punitive damages (damages to punish the company). He lost his case but Dennys later decided to make bigger seats available.

Seating does seem to cause quite a problem for those at the higher end of the weight spectrum. Companies providing seating for the public or their employees need to consider the size of their seats, to reduce the risk of humiliating their clients and staff.

Relationships - is there a weight effect?

There has not been much research into the effect of weight on relationships. The work that is documented tends to suggest that any negative effect of extra weight is felt more by women, than men. Among college undergraduates who were asked about their dating history in the USA, it was found that those who were overweight were less likely to be dating. If they were dating, they were less likely to be satisfied with their relationship. Nearly a third of the students in an exclusive relationship had been told to lose or gain weight by a partner (or had told the partner to gain or lose weight). Not surprisingly, those women told to lose weight were less satisfied with their relationship than other women. Whereas women were equally likely to have been told to lose or gain weight, men were more likely have been told to gain weight.

Personal advertisements of larger women looking for a dating partner have a more positive response when there is no weight description. Where there is a description, "full figured" or stating height and weight, are viewed more positively than the terms "obese", "overweight" or "fat".

The trouble with some studies is that because they are often done with groups of students asked to evaluate a hypothetical situation, it seems likely that they will resort to judging on stereotypes more than would happen in a real life situation. For instance, when students were asked by Eunice Chen (University of Washington) to rate drawings of potential sexual partners in order of preference (from a choice of healthy, amputee, obese, wheelchair user, history of suicide attempts and mental illness and history of curable sexually-transmitted disease who practiced safe sex) the category that students rated highest was "healthy" and the lowest category was "obese". The results were the same for both male and female students, although the men ranked the obese person even lower. Of course, in real life, the choice to date someone is not just based on a drawing. Many other factors (such as personality and interests) will be taken into account, so the relevance to the larger person and their relationships is questionable - although it does highlight the extent of the stigma associated with excess weight.

In adolescents, the dating record for larger boys was found to be the same as for normal weight boys. Among the girls, the larger girls were less likely to have dated than their peers. Girls were more willing to date a larger boy but boys were more concerned with the physical appearance of their partner. However, this type of study was done using anonymous questionnaires that also required the students to fill in their own height and weight. Unless adolescents have changed a lot since I was young, I think the tendency would be to feel that the questions were intrusive, and the temptation to give a false recording of weight or dating record would be quite high. In any case, most people tend to underestimate their weight and overestimate their own height.

In practice, the larger person should probably take no notice of this research on relationships and size - because if a person is going to adversely judge you on the basis of your physical characteristics, then quite obviously they are not worth bothering with. I am reminded of a comment made on TV recently by Sarah Millican (comedienne) who said that she was told by a male colleague that she was "actually quite attractive" and "if she lost two stone they could probably go out on a date". Her reply was "Only if the two stone that I lost was my head."

Children with weight problems

Gina Score was 14 years old when she was sent to a state juvenile detention camp in the USA, in 1999. She had been stealing small sums of money, from school lockers and her parents, to buy food. An intelligent girl, who liked writing poetry, she had paid most of the money back. At 5ft 4" tall she was 16 stone (224lbs/102kg) and found the camp regime, which was devised by a former marine, physically difficult. One hot and humid day, she was forced to begin a walk/run of nearly 3 miles. After falling behind, she was prodded and cajoled by camp staff until she collapsed. She was pale, frothing at the mouth and had purple lips. The instructors laughed and left her lying on the ground in the hot sun for 4 hours, whilst they sat drinking sodas and accusing her of faking. She died of organ failure.

In England, Kelly Yeomans aged 13, died after taking an overdose in 1997. She had been tormented about her weight by bullies at school and gangs of children yelled insults and threw stones, butter and eggs at her house, for several consecutive nights. She told her parents that she "couldn't take it any more".

These are the most extreme examples of weight-related bullying, but the effect of bullying or teasing on children cannot be overestimated. Although unrelated to weight issues, a study of 28 school shootings in the USA, found that most of the student shooters had been victims of severe teasing, which was often homophobic or critical of masculinity.

Around a third of obese youths say that they have been a victim of bullying or teasing. It can be in the form of verbal abuse, physical violence, social exclusion, being ignored or being the target of rumours. Children as young as 3 years old start to have a negative attitude towards larger people. By the age of 7-12 years, they are more likely to describe the obese as, "lazy, less happy and less attractive".

Even though more of us are becoming larger over recent years, this does not mean that because the problem is more common we are becoming more tolerant of size. In fact, the reverse seems to be happening. In 1961, children aged 11 were asked to rank pictures of children in order of which they would like to be friends with them. The pictures included a normal weight child with no disabilities, a child in a wheelchair, a child on crutches, a child with a missing hand, a child with a facial disfigurement and an obese child. The obese child was rated as least preferred to be a friend. A repeat of this experiment 25 years later by Dr Janet Latner (University of Hawaii) found that the obese child was still last in order of preference, but the distance between the average rankings of the highest and lowest ranked pictures had increased substantially.

Teachers can also give larger children a hard time at school. In a study in the USA, a fifth of secondary school teachers thought that the obese were "untidy, less likely to succeed in school, more emotional and more likely to have family problems". A substantial 43% believed that "most people feel uncomfortable when they associate with obese people". P.E. teachers seem to be the most strongly prejudiced against their larger pupils. Other studies have shown that obese adolescents who are bullied by other pupils, or receive negative remarks from teachers about their sporting abilities, are less likely to participate in sport and they try to avoid P.E. lessons.

Children may pick up from television some of their attitudes towards their larger colleagues. A survey of 6 year old boys found that the more television they watched, the greater the likelihood that they would negatively stereotype a larger woman, as television portrays thinness as the ideal shape for women. Children adopt fat stereotypes as do adults and perhaps surprisingly both overweight and non-overweight people are equally likely to have the same negative views.

What is the effect of this teasing or bullying on the larger child? It seems that around the age of 10 there is generally little difference in the self-esteem between normal weight and obese children. By the age of 13 or 14, there can be a significant lowering of self-esteem in the larger child. This can be manifest as loneliness, sadness or nervousness, and when poor self-esteem does occur, there is more chance of the child drinking or smoking. This is by no means universal. It is thought that when the parents are accepting of the child's weight and they are not critical about it, this can help maintain the child's self-esteem. Children who blame themselves for their weight problem are more likely to have a lower self-esteem, so it is important that they should know that the weight problem is not their fault.

Some people will try to justify criticising larger children in the mistaken belief that it will motivate them to lose weight. However, the evidence is that generally the reverse happens and they eat more, refuse to diet and get heavier.

Problems in children associated with weight, such as low self-esteem, are more common in older girls and in those whose weight is at the higher end of the weight spectrum. They tend to be most dissatisfied with their bodies. At its most extreme, teasing of adolescents about excess weight can be accompanied by depressive symptoms and thinking about suicide, as well as low self-esteem. This is most likely when the child is experiencing teasing about their weight from their family, as well as other children. It is the extent of the teasing that causes these problems, which have little relationship to the actual weight of the child. Parents most likely to give the larger child a difficult time are, statistically, fathers with a higher education and a high salary and parents who feel their own appearance is important. Parents often do not know how to help their children and they feel guilty that they might be to blame for the weight problem.

How can parents help their children? It seems that they need to avoid criticising or teasing about weight and they should let the child know that it is not their fault. They should avoid criticising other overweight people in front of their children and not refer to fat as "bad". Children can think that this means that fat people are bad. Overweight children get less friendship nominations than normal weight children (3.4 versus 4.8) in surveys of children age 13-18, who were asked to nominate friends. However, children of all weights get more nominations if they watch less television and participate in school clubs or sports clubs. Helping the larger child to develop some club memberships, cutting down on TV, and removing it from the child's bedroom could help. Problems such as depression and low self-esteem are not automatically associated with excess weight in children. Having a supportive and positive family can help protect children from developing these problems.

A small puppet program has been tried out in primary schools giving the message, "not to tease others" and "be a good friend", to promote greater acceptance of various body shapes. Lori Irving (Washington State University) reported that this had some success.

Of course, the first port of call in helping your child should be to have a chat with your family doctor, who should be able to at least tell you whether your child is clinically overweight or obese or not. If they are not able to help much, you could ask to see a dietician or paediatrician who is sympathetic to the problems of larger children. You would want to talk about the issue sensitively if your child is present, to avoid making them feel at all stigmatised.

Do check with your doctor that your child actually has a problem before worrying. Many adults think that they have a weight problem, whereas they are quite within the boundaries of what is medically considered to be a healthy normal weight. If your child is in the normal weight range for his/her height and age, they probably don't have a problem. If the medical advice is that your child is overweight or obese, then ask for help from a professional who is sympathetic and will support the child and not make them feel worse or stigmatised. I am loath to give much general advice here for children, as I think that their health is so important that they deserve the individual attention of a dietician or doctor who has an interest in the problem.

How do people cope with discrimination?

If you have a weight problem, how have you coped with the discrimination that you have encountered? Particularly if you are a larger woman, it will have been difficult to avoid.

Various ways in which people cope with the stigma that can be associated with weight have been described, but there doesn't seem to be much evidence yet as to which methods work the best and for whom. Some of these coping strategies seem to be more positive than others. A poor way of coping would be to behave in the way that the prejudiced person expects, for instance - "OK, you think I'm lazy, so I will be". This isn't likely to enhance self-esteem. Around 80% of larger people report eating more food as a way of coping, when they feel that they have been stigmatised. Blaming oneself for the problem or avoiding situations, tends to be done by those who are naturally more anxious and pessimistic, and probably leads to further distress. In particular, larger women who subscribe to the ethic that, "you get what you deserve in life", tend to be more distressed about their weight. Many will cope with stigmatisation by trying to lose weight, or pretending to try and lose weight, to reduce the social pressure. Some will even resort to surgery.

Men are more likely to confront the person who is prejudiced against their size. In one small study, three quarters of the men said that they used witty replies or rejoinders when subject to stigmatisation. Only a very small proportion reported being physically aggressive towards the insulting person.

Avoiding going out in public and avoiding mirrors is very common among the largest people and probably doesn't help as a long term strategy for managing a weight problem. Whereas avoiding people might deal with the problem in the short term, in the long term it might reduce social skills.

Those who have a personality that is generally optimistic might tend to use more active coping strategies to cope with stigma. One approach might be to value other attributes about oneself to diminish the importance of weight. People who have been large from childhood may be particularly assertive and friendly in social situations. Joining an organisation, such as the National Association to Advance Fat Acceptance, if you are in the USA, can help some people cope by celebrating weight. Trying to head off unpleasant remarks when they crop up in conversation may also be a strategy worth following.

Self-acceptance and positive self-talk (talking to oneself silently or out loud for motivation or encouragement) may help if you are experiencing prejudice. One study, where people were shown how to challenge stereotypes and be more assertive, found an improvement in self-esteem of the participants. They also became less restricted in their daily activities and were less subject to depressed mood.

Dr Leanne Joanisse (McMaster University) interviewed a small sample of larger people to find out how they coped with the stigma of weight. She found that there was a variety of methods used, and sometimes people would progress from one to another. Although she was unable to present evidence as to which was the most effective strategy, her findings were nevertheless interesting. She found that some people would be passive and try not to show that they were upset, whilst others would be more active in challenging prejudice.

One of the ways of coping with insults was to retaliate - such as sarcastically complimenting the insulting person on their good visual acuity. Some of the people would just flatly refuse to allow their families to discuss their weight, and would refuse to stand on their doctor's scales, if they did not want to. Others would be physically more aggressive - one man described how his strategy was to throw chocolate milk. When a man in a passing car called him a "big fat slob" and made "blowfish cheeks" at him, he threw his chocolate milk through the car window. He estimated that he had had to throw chocolate milk at people around fifteen times in the last eight years. This chocolate milk approach I really would not recommend - apart from being a waste of milk, it runs the risk that you might be physically attacked or cause a traffic accident.

Adopting a striking appearance, by wearing bright clothes and dyeing the hair bright red and so forth, was a strategy used successfully by some, particularly in the entertainment field. People that seemed to suffer least from size-ism were those who were secure in themselves and what they had to offer people. They considered that being large was "just part of me". These people tended to be the ones that had received unconditional love from at least one other person when they were growing up. Maybe it helped protect them from prejudice. Others were described as "enlightened" and these had often reached the age of around 45, after a lifetime of struggling with their weight. They were resigned to it, and thought that they had always been big and that they were just going to have to live with it.

There were some positive aspects to being big - a teacher described using his size to impose his authority on the class.

Some felt that they were more sympathetic to the sufferings of others (such as the disabled) because they had been through so much themselves.

In the absence of much good evidence as to which strategies for coping with prejudice are the best, it seems that you need to make your own judgment, depending on the extent of the problem and what suits your own personality. In general, being assertive without being aggressive, or ignoring the prejudiced person if possible, as well as seeking out support from sympathetic people, may be among the better strategies. Cultivating a friendly and outgoing personality and trying not to avoid going out, is probably also better than avoiding people and situations. Obviously, don't blame yourself for your weight problem. It is, of course, a real shame that this prejudice exists and hopefully in the future attitudes towards the weight-challenged will change, so that any consideration of how to cope with discrimination will become irrelevant.

Chapter 7: Do you have a weight problem - if so what should you do about it?

Check if you have a weight problem

Many people who think that they are overweight are actually a normal weight. The first thing to do, is to check your weight against a healthy weight chart, such as is shown on the next page. (1 stone = 14lbs, if you are used to thinking of weight in lbs only.)

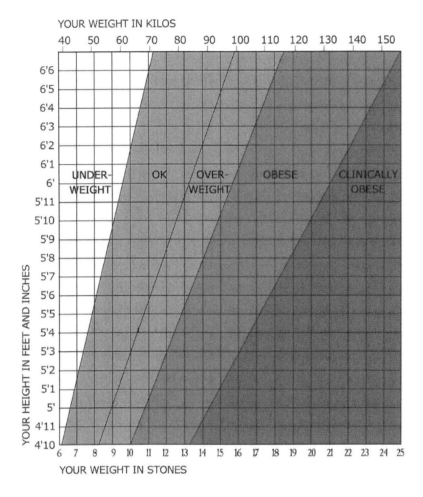

YOUR WEIGHT IN KILOS

YOUR HEIGHT IN FEET AND INCHES

YOUR WEIGHT IN STONES

This is a guide to weight, based on height. Look at the weight appropriate to your height. If, for instance, you are 5ft 4" tall, the maximum healthy weight is around 10 stone 5lbs (145lbs/66kg). If you are 6ft tall, the maximum healthy weight is around 13 stone 3lbs (185lbs/84kg). If you are under these weights, then you are in the healthy weight category, or the underweight category. If you are over the healthy weight, then you are overweight, or if the weight is more significant, you will then be classified as obese. The very highest category, at the top of the obese range, is sometimes described as very obese, morbidly obese or clinically obese.

What if you are not overweight?

If you are not above the healthy weight limit for your height, or even approaching it, but are firmly in the healthy weight zone, then you are not overweight and your weight is normal. You may not feel normal but this is largely due to images in the media where, particularly for women, underweight is considered normal. Humans are designed to have a layer of fat under the skin and by the time the age of eighteen is reached, a normal boy has 12% of his weight as fat tissue and a normal girl has 24% of her weight as fat tissue. In girls, this is particularly deposited on the hips, breasts and thighs and is completely normal. There is nothing desirable or healthy about being underweight.

If you are in the healthy weight category, particularly in the middle of it, there is probably little need to be concerned about your weight. Eating healthy food and making sure that you are not too sedentary might well be enough to stop a weight problem developing. There is, as we have previously mentioned, a genetic component to weight. If your relatives are all overweight or obese, then you might want to weigh yourself monthly and start to take corrective action when you approach the top of the healthy weight limit.

If you are a healthy weight and your weight is normal, then life is too short to spend time worrying about a non-existent weight problem.

Checked the chart - what do you do?

If there is one message that comes out clearly from looking at the research into weight problems, it is that there is a great variation between people in how they can effectively manage their weight. If you are overweight, you need to find an individual strategy that works for you. You are aiming for gradual and sustained weight loss, which will be permanent.

Before making an individual plan, I would suggest that it would be worth spending some time considering your own personal circumstances. If you have read the rest of this book, you may already have some ideas for strategies that might work for you. If you need more guidance I would suggest you first consider several different areas of your life which relate to weight problems, starting with your genes and childhood.

Genes, childhood and upbringing

In the future, genetic tests for genes associated with obesity will probably become freely available, but for now, the best way to judge your genetic inheritance might be to get out some family photograph albums. Look at the body size of your blood relatives - parents, grandparents, brothers, sisters and children. What weight are they? If they are all lean and athletic, you can be encouraged that you might find returning to a healthy weight less arduous than many. On the other hand, if you are looking at a series of rotund relatives - well, you are more likely to have "survivor genes" that help conserve fat for a state of famine. You can though, take heart that one of the reasons for your weight problem is obvious. It is not greed or lack of willpower. Your genes are attempting to pile the weight on. This does not mean that you will not be able to take the weight off (you will) but it does mean that you can stop blaming yourself.

Whilst you have the family photos out, look at pictures of yourself pre-school, at your first school and in your early teens. Were you a normal weight lean child, or was there a weight problem then? If you were a normal weight child, it may mean that you will be able to lose weight more easily than those that had a significant weight problem throughout their childhood. If you were obviously overweight as a child it might be a little more difficult to lose the weight but it is still entirely possible, though you might need to monitor things more carefully than someone who was a normal weight child.

What was family life like when you were growing up, with regards to food? Where was the food eaten and if it was at home, who did the shopping and cooking? Often, behaviour patterns set by adults are followed by children. Harriette Snoek (Radboud University) found that four or five year old children, when buying food at a miniature toy supermarket and playing at being "mother buying food for the family", choose different foods to buy. The overweight children choose food of higher calorie value than that selected by normal weight children.

Have your food shopping and eating habits been an extension

of what was eaten in your childhood home? Did the family home tend to eat healthy fresh food or was there a bias towards high fat and processed food? How important was food when you were growing up? Was there more of an "eat to live" or "live to eat" attitude? Was feeding people thought to be synonymous with caring for them? Were celebrations always marked by meals or food, or were there other ways of celebrating?

Attitudes to eating and weight can be adopted when young. What was the attitude of other family members to their own weight and to your weight? Were they unconcerned, or did you hear a constant barrage of self-criticism from a family member who was always trying to diet? Were the family unconcerned with your weight or were you either encouraged to "eat everything on the plate", so you could "have dessert", or criticised if you ate too much, or for being overweight? Was food referred to as "good" or "bad" food and was guilt associated with eating cakes or sweet foods?

Food and our attitude to it can be an emotional minefield and identifying where your own attitude to food comes from can help when you plan how to tackle a weight problem.

What is your present attitude to food?

Your present attitude to food and eating might still be the same as the attitude you had when growing up, or have been changed by subsequent life experiences. It is difficult to give blanket advice in a book, when the question is so individual, but there are some areas that you might want to consider if you are having difficulty clarifying your own reaction to food. It might be worth considering whether your attitude to food is uncontrolled, emotional or restrained, and whether your own thinking about food is dichotomous (black and white) or more relaxed.

Is your eating uncontrolled?

For instance, you could ask yourself these questions:

- Does the smell of frying onions or steak mean that you find it difficult to keep from eating, even if you are full? (yes/no)

- Once you start eating, do you then find it difficult to stop? (yes/no)
- Are you generally hungry most of the time? (yes/no)
- If you see tempting food, do you get so hungry that you have to eat it straight away? (yes/no)
- If you are with someone who is eating, do you have to join them, as it makes you feel hungry too? (yes/no)
- Do you always eat everything on your plate? (yes/no)
- Do you eat large amounts when you are not hungry? (yes/no)

If you have answered "yes" to many of these questions, then there may be an element to your eating which is uncontrolled. This does not mean that it is your fault (or that you are greedy) but it is useful to recognise how you behave towards food in order to successfully change your eating patterns. You could tell yourself that because others are eating, you do not have to join them, and take a moment to decide whether you are hungry or not. Even if you have been brought up to clear your plate because "starving children in Africa would be glad of that food", finishing some food when you are not hungry will not help a food shortage in Africa at all. Stopping eating when you are full is a better attitude to try and adopt. If you tend towards uncontrolled eating, then avoiding places and situations where tempting food is readily available, when you are not hungry, is advisable.

As I have already mentioned, this sort of uncontrolled eating is not your fault. There is a genetic component to this type of eating. Studies of twins by Kaisu Keskitalo (University of Helsinki) have found that the heritability of uncontrolled eating is 45-70% of the trait. Uncontrolled eating is characterised by a genetic and environmental associated liking for salty-and-fatty foods, such as fried potatoes, chips, salty snacks, pizza, hamburgers, fish in batter and fried foods.

If this describes your type of eating (if you eat in an uncontrolled way, and have inherited a liking for the salty-fatty food types) it does not mean that you are doomed to eat large amounts of greasy food, in an uncontrolled fashion. It just means that you can use this information to recognise the problem. This is useful when you come to decide which steps you might take to lose weight.

Do you eat in response to emotion?

- Do you eat when you feel sad? (yes/no)
- Do you eat when anxious? (yes/no)
- Do you eat when lonely? (yes/no)

Of course, you will have realised that answering "yes" to these questions implies that there is an emotional component to your eating. Again, there is a tendency for this emotional eating to be inherited to some extent, with Keskitalo putting the heritability at between 9% and 45%. Emotional eating is also associated with a genetic liking for "sweet-and-fatty" food, such as ice-cream, chocolate, sweet pastry and sweet desserts. Emotional eaters eat more snack food.

If this applies to you, recognising that it is happening will be helpful as you can then go on to plan how to address the problem. If, for instance, you are eating because you are anxious about something, consider what else you could do to deal with the situation and reduce your own anxiety levels. Could you confront the problem and sort it out, or confide in a friend or get help with the problem? If you are an emotional eater, taking a moment before you head to the kitchen in times of stress, sadness or loneliness, and thinking about what else you could do to alleviate the problem might help.

Are you a restrained eater?

- Do you avoid some foods because they make you fat? (yes/no)
- Do you have small helpings to keep your weight down? (yes/no)
- Do you eat less than you would like? (yes/no)
- Do you avoid stockpiling your favourite foods or foods you think might make you put on weight? (yes/no)

If you have answered "yes" to most of these questions, then

you are probably tending to consciously monitor, or restrain, your eating. There is a school of thought that associates these restrained eating thinking patterns with a tendency to eat large amounts of food episodically. The rigid restraint path chosen becomes too difficult and breaks down, leading to episodes of uncontrolled or binge eating. The restrained trait is inherited to a certain degree (26%-63%). Whereas some degree of restraint in the food arena is obviously a good thing (otherwise we would just eat everything in sight) it is possible that excessive restraint can lead to eating large amounts when the restraint breaks down, which then leads to weight gain. It is the degree of restraint which is important to the individual.

In adults, restrained eating is associated with eating more healthy food, such as green vegetables and less chips or sugar. However, in teenagers and young adults, it is associated with less high fat food consumption, and there is no particular association with healthy eating.

It has to be said that "restraint" as a concept when applied to eating habits is of questionable scientific validity, as you would think that those people who have high scores on restraint scales would tend to eat less. Some of the studies of dietary restraint showed that the restraint scores did not correlate well with the quantity of food eaten. For instance, Eric Stice (University of Texas) persuaded female students to taste three types of cookies (chocolate chip, peanut and sugar) telling them that they were studying the relationship between mood and the taste of cookies. They were actually looking to see whether the students' restraint scores correlated with how many cookies they ate. Each student was given three plates of freshly baked cookies and told to eat as many as she liked, as they had to bake fresh ones for the next volunteer. Hidden cameras watched them and one student was excluded from the results as she was seen to tip a plate of cookies into her backpack. The results showed that the restraint scores did not relate to the amount of calories eaten.

Similarly, people eating in a fast food restaurant were covertly watched to see what they ate and then asked to fill in dietary restraint scales. There was only a weak correlation (which was not statistically significant) with relation to the number of calories actually consumed. At this point, the researchers even contemplated covertly watching people in their own homes to see if what they were eating correlated to the scores they got of dietary restraint. Fortunately, they were unable to find an ethically acceptable method of collecting the information. Further tests, using double labelled water (which gives an actual indication of the amount of calories consumed over a two week period) did not find any good correlation with scores on scales of dietary restraint.

In the past, restraint scales had been shown to correlate with the amount of food eaten, but this was self-reported intake and this type of recording is notoriously unreliable. It seems to be particularly unreliable in those who score highly on dietary restraint scales. Some surveys have even shown that people who have high scores of restraint tend to go on to put on weight. It might be that scales of dietary restraint are assessing relative, rather than actual, dietary restriction. People with high scores are eating less than they would like and think they are being restrained, whereas in fact they have not cut back enough to lose weight, or are still eating enough to put on weight. One person's idea of restraint might be another person's idea of a large meal.

How does this debate about restraint affect you? Well, as no one is covertly watching what you are eating, you can afford to be honest with yourself. We all have to have some degree of restraint or we would eat everything in sight, but is the degree of restraint becoming a problem? Do you, for instance, try and be restrained all day, sticking to a low calorie regime, to find that by evening you become so hungry that you give up all restraint? You then have a huge evening meal, and end up eating far more than you would have done had you not been restrained in the first place. In this case, the restraint is going too far and in effect might cause weight gain.

Do you exhibit dichotomous thinking?

- You're either my friend or my enemy (agree/disagree)
- You're either a winner or a loser (agree/disagree)
- People are either good or bad (agree/disagree)
- I prefer competitions to have clear results (agree/disagree)
- You are either fat or you are thin (agree/disagree)

- Food is either "good" or "bad" food (agree/disagree)
- I'm either a "success" or a "failure"(agree/disagree)

Of course, if you agree with these sorts of sentiments, your thinking probably tends to be dichotomous (see chapter 5 for an explanation of dichotomous thinking). If you think in this rigid way it can be more difficult to keep weight off. This tendency might be something you need to consider, when you plan how to manage a weight problem. Adding shades of grey into your thinking with relation to food, eating and body image, and not seeing everything as "black or white" can be helpful. Of course, whether you want to change your way of thinking in relation to other areas of life is a different matter, and one of personal preference. Dichotomous thinking has been linked to conservative political attitudes. It might also be partly cultural. Atsushi Oshio (Waseda University) found that Russian women had a greater tendency to dichotomous thinking than Japanese women.

Having rigid ideas and rules about food can perhaps lead to binge eating or over-indulgence when the rules are broken, leading to weight gain.

If you think that you might suffer from dichotomous thinking in relation to food, then modifying your language so it is less dichotomous can help change thinking patterns. Instead of saying, "oh dear, I've eaten a huge bar of chocolate, I'm really fat", which tends to lead to thinking, "I'm really fat anyway, I might as well have a pudding", modifying the language to, "I've eaten a bar of chocolate, it was 100g (3.5oz) which won't help my weight but it is not the end of the world", might lead to thoughts such as, "I'll just make sure I don't buy a large bar in future", or "I'll have a small dinner and that will help offset some of the calories".

Considering attitude to food can help normalise thoughts about food, which will be helpful to anyone with a weight problem. If any of the above categories seems familiar to you, then you can use that information to plan weight management.

Women are more likely to exhibit restrained eating or emotional eating, whereas men are slightly more likely to eat foods which are both salty-and-fatty. Younger people are more likely to have uncontrolled eating and older people more likely to have restrained eating. You might fall into one of these categories more than others, or exhibit behaviours across categories, but considering your answers might give you more insight into how and why you eat. People are all different and these differences are important when considering lifestyle changes. Trying to normalise your attitude to food, if you are a long term "dieter" can be helpful because many such people tend to categorise food as "good" or "bad" food, depending on its calorie content. They feel virtuous if they eat the good food and guilty if they eat the bad. After a while, some people just overeat because they feel they are "going to fail anyway". Getting the attitude to food back to normal can lead to normalisation of eating patterns with regular meals of moderate portions. This leads to becoming more in-tune with the body and eating when hungry.

On the other hand, if you never exhibit uncontrolled or emotional eating, you have only normal levels of restraint and your attitudes are generally flexible, perhaps losing weight will be easier for you than for others and this is encouraging.

Who do you live with?

Years ago, I had a job that included screening patients who were awaiting surgery for obesity, to make sure that they had no psychiatric conditions before the operation went ahead. On introducing myself to the patient, I was careful to explain that all the patients had a pre-op check, to make sure that there were no problems with their mental health that could be affecting their weight. People can incorrectly assume that just having to talk to a psychiatrist implies that someone thinks they have a mental health problem. I remember explaining this to one large gentleman in his fifties and he found this very amusing. When he finished laughing he said, "No, it's just my wife, she's a really good cook!" Subsequent questioning confirmed that he did not have any evidence of a mental health disorder, and his wife's cooking sounded very tempting. She really liked baking, and he described her pies, cakes and so forth in glowing terms. Sometimes the reasons for a weight problem are obvious. You did not need to delve deep to see that a man who liked to eat, surrounded by quantities of appetising high fat food, is likely to put on weight.

Of course, there is the separate question of his relationship with his wife. If someone is cooking so much that their spouse has to undergo surgery, because of the problem that they have helped to create, you do wonder about their own motivation and relationship with food. I am not suggesting that the spouse was deliberately overfeeding her husband (after all, no one is force-fed) but preparing food for the family can be viewed as an expression of caring or loving the family. When this is overdone, it is possible that excess weight could be a problem.

Some time ago, a colleague I was working with got married and invited us to the wedding. In the months following the event, my colleague, who was a normal weight when he got married, began to noticeably and rapidly put on weight. Remarks were made to me by my boss such as, "marriage seems to agree with him, he's putting on a lot of weight", but it did not seem to be any of our business. However, one lunch time he brought the subject up himself and said that he was concerned about the amount of weight he seemed to be piling on since he got married. It transpired that his wife would present him with a huge array of delicious Asian dishes in the evening, as she would get home from work and start cooking. If he did not eat everything she would be upset and think he did not like her food, so he felt obliged to tuck in. I asked if she was gaining weight (she had seemed quite slender at the wedding) but he said no, she wouldn't eat the food herself, she would just watch him eat. The obvious solution was to talk to her about it, point out that he was getting bigger and suggest that although her food was lovely, perhaps she could cook a bit less or eat some herself?

It is probably worth considering how the attitude of those you live with affects your own eating habits. If someone else is usually buying or preparing food and this is part of your weight problem, then involving them and getting them onside will be an important part of any change towards healthier eating. I am not suggesting you apportion blame to your spouse or relatives for a weight problem. Sometimes people can confuse love and food and think that if they are not feeding their family large amounts of delicious food, then it is a sign that they do not love them.

Cooking for family can be difficult, on the one hand it is seen as a demonstration of "caring" behaviour, but if taken to excess can be detrimental. If one or more of the family members have a significant weight problem, then it is worth taking a step back and considering how the actions of the other family members might be contributing to the problem - not to allocate blame, but to work together to find a solution.

What are you eating?

If you have a digital or phone camera you could go straight away and open the fridge and food cupboards and take a picture of what you see, before you have time to think about it. Then collect your recent grocery receipts if you have them - if you shop online this is easy to find in your old shopping orders. Then write down everything you have eaten in the last twenty-four hours. Include any alcoholic drinks or drinks that have higher calorie content such as milkshakes, smoothies and fizzy drinks. Do all this straight away before you have time to manipulate your cupboards and you will have an honest snapshot of your diet. You do not have to show it to anyone else. I am not going to suggest that you keep a food diary, because just the act of keeping one will alter what you are eating and you want a fair reflection of what you are actually consuming.

Have a look at the information you have gathered. What proportion of the food you are consuming is unadulterated healthy food such as fruit, vegetables, lean meat, poultry or fish? What proportion is of pre-prepared ready meals and less healthy foods such as cakes, biscuits, sweets or fizzy drinks? What are you faced with when you open the fridge? Is it full of fresh vegetables and salad, with maybe a chicken, or does it contain microwave meals, ready-made desserts and cakes and processed meats, such as sausages? What did you actually eat in the last 24 hours? Were there plenty of vegetables and healthy foods, or was it mostly deep fried and processed food?

I would suggest you then make a list of your ten most favourite and ten least favourite foods. When you come to make a plan to adjust your lifestyle and eating patterns, including some of the favourites might make it easier to stick to the new regime. There is no point trying to make meal plans which include foods that you particularly dislike.

Medical conditions

Do you have any medical conditions? When deciding on lifestyle changes it is in any case a good idea to check with your doctor that there will be no adverse effect on health, and that the changes you are planning will have a positive health effect. If you have conditions such as diabetes, you are likely to need expert dietary advice and the health service should provide this. If you are young, you will also be in particular need of medical help as any dietary changes you make need to take into account that you are still growing. You need to make sure you don't cut down on food too much and still have adequate nutrients for growth. If you are pregnant you need to get plenty of good nutrition and any changes you are thinking of making should definitely be cleared with your doctor or midwife. In any case, there are certain foods that pregnant women need to avoid and they should inform you of these. If you are subject to binge eating, self-induced vomiting or laxative abuse, in a mistaken attempt to control weight, you should certainly seek medical help, as all these practices can have serious adverse medical consequences and should be avoided.

If you see your family doctor and he/she agrees that you have a weight problem, particularly in the obese range, they might also suggest blood tests for glucose (sugar), lipids (fats), thyroid function, liver function and other metabolic tests, which will help in an assessment of your situation.

How much exercise do you do?

Do you do any sporting exercise - football, golf, swimming and so forth? If you are doing it less than once a week it is unlikely to make much difference long term to the amount of calories you are using up. If you regularly play and enjoy sport, then that is a plus if you are trying to get down to a healthy weight. If you do not have a sport, is there anything you would enjoy? It is more likely to help reduce your weight if you are male, so if you are an overweight man, taking up some regular sport is a good idea. Of course, you need to choose something that is age and health appropriate. Golf, walking, or gentle swimming, will be much better for an overweight 45 year old than, say, taking up squash or other extreme forms of exercise.

Apart from sport, generally moving around more in our daily living is where most of the difference can be made to use up more calories. This is the more important area to look at really. Few people have the time or inclination to take up hard physical training.

How much do you move at work and home? If you can afford it, you might wish to buy a cheap pedometer. You can get one for around £15 ($25).This is a small instrument which you clip to your belt and by detecting movement of the hips, it can add up the number of steps you have taken each day. If you calibrate it to your step size, it can work out the distance you walk each day. I would recommend you wear it for at least a week, noting down the distance you walk each day and whether there is much of a difference between weekends and weekdays. Try to just do what you normally do, as this will give you a proper baseline reading. Check it is accurate, some of the cheaper pedometers will count going over a bump in the car as a step.

Also, think about what proportion of the day you spend sitting. Are most of your journeys on foot, or by car or bus? Do you take the stairs or the lift at work? Does your work involve exercise? A postal delivery person will be getting more exercise than a call centre worker.

This information should help you plan how you can increase the amount of activity you do, to help lose weight. Some guidelines suggest that around 6,000 steps a day on a pedometer is good for health, and 10,000 for weight loss, but you are probably best finding out what your normal number is, then deciding how much you want to aim to increase it. This depends on your state of health and age. You should consult a doctor about the rate of increase, but starting at a 10% increase, if you are a fit healthy young adult, might be a reasonable first step.

Make a plan

By now, you might have some ideas about how you can manage your weight problem. An approach tailored to the individual is most likely to produce long term success in losing weight and keeping it off. You might already have seen ideas that are particularly appropriate - but if you still need some direction, you could make a plan incorporating all the areas associated with weight loss that are relevant to you.

If you have read the preceding chapters and gathered all the data you can find on your genetic disposition, eating and exercise habits, you are now in a good position to make an individual plan to reduce your weight to a healthy level and to maintain it there. Fitting the changes you need to your own individual requirements means that you are much more likely to be successful in keeping weight off in the long term, than if you follow a one-size-fits-all diet of the sort that regularly crops up in the January magazines and newspapers.

While we are on the subject, I do believe that New Year's Day is the worst time to make a resolution to lose weight or attempt anything difficult. I once worked a New Year's Day in general practice and I was astonished at the calls I was getting. (This was before the new medical contract, when family doctors provided a 24 hour service, instead of the ridiculous office hours service that has now been adopted in the UK.) Anyhow, the calls I got on New Year's Day were most unusual. Generally you might get calls to visit for a range of medical problems. On New Year's Day I was busy making lots of visits, but they were all emotional problems, family arguments with suspected overdose and generalised depression or anxiety problems. The next day, I described to the partners what had happened and they apologised and said they should have warned me that New Year's Day was always like that. I think it might be something to do with having to face a New Year, and having this artificial calendar date when it is conventional to assess how your life is going and to plan changes. There is also the prospect of having to cope with going back to work after a long break.

So when you are making a plan, try not to start on New Year's Day. Any other day might be better. Try not to make the changes so extreme that you are not going to be able to sustain them. Think of the long term and not a crash diet approach. There is no perfect diet that will fit everyone. Although it is tempting to follow the fashion in this matter and embrace whichever diet is now promising fantastic results, with celebrity endorsement, you are more likely to be successful in losing and maintaining weight loss if the changes you make suit yourself and relate to the kind of food you like to eat. Make changes which are not too extreme and are sustainable.

Remember also, that there is a lot of evidence that losing weight is relatively easy in the short term, and extremely difficult in the long term. For this reason, making changes that promote a healthy lifestyle are probably what you should be aiming for. If you cannot get down to a normal weight, you can improve the situation by eating healthy food and doing enough exercise (appropriate to your age and gender) as it is better to be "large and fit" rather than "large and unfit".

The areas you might want to cover in the plan are:

- Goal weight
- Personal food environment
- Changing attitudes to food
- Exercise and activity
- Social support
- Weight monitoring
- Coping with weight stigma

Do you want a "goal weight"?

Many people like to have an idea of the weight that they would like to achieve. There is some evidence that it is easier to achieve proximal (nearer) goals than it is to achieve goals that are further away. If you need to lose a lot of weight, then stopping the weight increasing might be your first aim, and then trying to reduce it to as near normal as possible (keeping in mind that any reduction will be helpful). If you can get, for instance, from being in the "obese" band of the weight graph, into the "overweight" band and stay there, then that is a significant achievement. Similarly, if you are in the "very obese" range, your first aim will probably be to stop more weight accumulating, then to get down to the "obese" range.

What is your ultimate aim? It is better to be realistic here. If you are just a few pounds overweight, then getting into the healthy weight band is a reasonable aim. Depending on your general build, you might prefer to be at the top end of the healthy weight range, or nearer the middle. I would suggest that any goal weight should certainly not be less than the middle of the healthy weight range. If you are in the "very obese" category, then setting a goal to get into the obese range, and then the overweight range and maintain that weight, might be as much as you can realistically manage. Certainly, it will put you in a much better position from the health point of view.

Johan Koeslag (Assoc. Professor of Physiology) argues that the "normal" weight of an 18 year old is not what a middle-aged person should be aiming for, and it is normal to add 20% more weight in middle-age. The average weight of both men and women at the age of 45 is 20% higher than it was at the age of 20 years - so perhaps your weight in your late teens is not something for which you need to aim.

The European Clinical Practice Guidelines state that weight loss objectives should be realistic, individualised and aimed at the long term. They suggest a practical aim might be a 5-15% weight loss, over a six month period, with a higher aim of 20% weight loss for those with a BMI of over 35. I think these guidelines should be taken as such, and finding a practical goal that suits you is probably the most important criteria.

Food - and changing your personal food environment

You now have evidence of what you are eating at present and perhaps from this you can see areas of your normal diet that are contributing to the weight problem. How to tackle this? Well, from the review of diets earlier in this book, there are many possible types of diets that have been described over the years and it might be that one of these, in particular, appeals to you. If so, check with your family doctor that it is safe for you to follow. If you don't have an inclination to follow a particular diet, then you might have noticed that most of the better diets have a lot of similarities. They tend to be based on consumption of unprocessed fresh food - in particular vegetables, fruit, cereals, pulses, wholegrain, lean meat, poultry, fish and normal dairy products from the lower fat part of the range. Making your first aim a healthy diet is a reasonable step for most people.

I would suggest that it might also be helpful to invest in a small booklet that gives the calorie and fat content of different foods. This is not so you can necessarily start counting fat or calories, but so that, if you are unfamiliar with nutritional values, you will be better able to identify healthy food that is naturally low in fat. (If you put "calorie and fat counter" into the search of Amazon or any other bookstore, you will find a selection of books. One small enough to fit in a pocket or bag might be best.)

From this point, it is difficult for me to say what is best for you as an individual, as we are all so varied in size and dietary preferences. I hope, from the following suggestions, you can pick out the ideas which will suit your needs. You might, for instance, have a particular need for social support and be considering joining one of the slimming groups available, but if you are undecided about how to tackle weight I think the "default" position is to go for a healthy diet. Certainly, from my reading of the available research, if I had a significant weight problem (and particularly in the obese or larger categories) this would be my first step. Predominately buying food that is unprocessed and fresh, and reducing the availability of processed, high fat food and fizzy drinks, would be a great first step.

What is a healthy diet? Trying to get a balanced diet, in general terms, means that your diet will consist of:

- One third of your food should be from the bread and cereals group (including rice, pasta and potatoes) equivalent to about six servings a day from this group.

- One third of your food should be vegetables and fruit. Preferably more vegetables than fruit, as they tend to be more nutritious (and cheaper).

- Of the rest, you should have 2 servings a day of protein containing foods such as meat, fish, poultry, eggs and pulses (such as beans). Also 2 servings of food from the milk and dairy group (to make sure you have enough calcium). Try to go more for milk, or yoghurt dairy that is naturally lower in fat (as opposed to products which are high fat, such as hard cheese). This leaves a small amount of space in the diet for fats, oils and sweets, which should be fairly minimal when trying to lose weight. It is difficult to be specific about the amount of fat needed, as this will vary between people depending on their size. A maximum total fat of 65g (2.3oz) a day is often suggested - however in practice this is not very helpful, as you can't easily measure all the fat in food. Removing visible fat from foods such as meat, and using cooking methods which do not use fat or only minimally (such as non-stick pans) is probably the best you can do.

A healthy diet is a good aim. Although counting calories or fat content of food can help you to educate yourself about which foods are healthiest, hopefully you should not need to do this long term once you have found a way of eating that works for you. Eating healthy food, stopping when you are no longer hungry and keeping the portions reasonable, rather than obsessing about food or weight, might be the best way forward for most people. However, if counting calories seems an attractive proposition to you, or if switching to a healthy balanced diet is not effective enough for your own particular weight problem, the European Clinical Practice Guidelines rule of thumb, is that you need to eat 25 calories per kg (2.2lbs) of body weight each day, in order to lose weight.

There is no way to avoid it but it is going to be a bit of a shock to the system at first, if you replace a diet of ready meals and convenience foods with "proper" food. If you are not used to cooking and you are faced with a fridge at the end of the day containing lots of vegetables and maybe some chicken, it will take time to develop skills that can make tasty food quickly. Personally, I am not that keen on cooking but there is no getting away from the fact that it is going to take a bit longer to cook, than it is to take a frozen pizza out of the freezer and put it in the oven. The plus side is that your food will probably taste much better, it will be more nutritious, and if you are cooking for a family it might well be cheaper than buying ready meals. You will probably find that shop bought ready meals begin to become unpalatable in comparison with home cooking. They often lack texture and have an amorphous quality that tends to occur in food that has been sitting in a box for a few days on a supermarket shelf.

Planning some of your meals in advance will be very helpful

from the shopping point of view, although after a while you should find it easier to know what to buy. If you do supermarket shopping, making a list and not adding any impulse buys (unless they come into the category of healthy, unprocessed and nutritious food) will help. Shopping online has some advantages, because you can see exactly what is in your shopping basket before you buy, and you know how much it is all going to cost. Before you order, review the list and ask yourself, is there anything there that is processed or pre-prepared, that I can do without or make myself? Actually going around the supermarket yourself will give you more exercise, but be careful as it requires a lot of discipline to stick to a list in a large store.

Your shopping should be based on lots of fresh vegetables and fruit (with more vegetables than fruit) lean meat, fish, poultry, eggs, low fat natural dairy products such as milk, cottage cheese and yoghurt, good bread, pasta, beans, lentils, rice, cereals (especially wholegrain), herbs and spices. If you can, avoid using butter too much. Instead use mustards, chutneys, jams and marmalade and so forth with bread, as it will cut down the fat content of your diet. Changing your personal food environment, so that high fat unhealthy food is no longer available, will cut down on the automatic consumption of these high calorie foods. Replacing the biscuit tin with a fruit bowl and making sure that only fresh unprocessed food is available, can be helpful. Foods to avoid buying include processed food, ready meals, ready-made cakes, sweets, biscuits and fizzy drinks. Most foods with over 10% fat content (10g per 100g) are unlikely to be helpful to those wanting to lose weight.

Other advice often given is to cook with only the minimum of fat and to remove all visible fat. For instance, with bacon, you can cook it on a rack in the oven over a tray, so the fat drips off, then cut off all the visible fat or use "medallions" of bacon. Boiled or poached eggs have less fat than those fried in oil and baked potatoes have less fat than roast - common sense stuff really.

If you can manage on healthy food but you think that you will need a small amount of something sweet in your eating plan to make it realistic for you to follow, then foods such as boiled sweets, marshmallows, meringues, plain pretzels, scones, Swiss rolls, whisked sponges or tea loaf (no butter in the ingredients) tend to be low in fat. However, you would not want to be eating large quantities of these items, as they are not particularly nutritious, and some have a large proportion of sugar in their ingredients.

If you generally eat food from other cultures, such as Asian food, then still sticking to the purchase of healthier items and cooking with less fat is possible. A book such as *Indian Cooking without Fat* by Mridula Baljekar, might be useful.

Eating out can be a problem and something you might need to consider. As well as the problems of automatic eating in company that we have already discussed, sticking to lower fat, less processed, menu choices is probably the best option - as is avoiding sauces that incorporate cream. Deep fried or fried food is also generally best avoided. Try and find something grilled or baked. In an Italian restaurant, pasta with a tomato sauce is better than with a cream sauce and the pizza toppings to avoid are sausage, pepperoni and cheese - whereas ham, chicken or vegetable toppings are fine. With salads, use the minimum of French type dressing and avoid mayonnaise dressings. In a curry house, plain rice with roast/grilled chicken (tandoori type) and vegetables will probably be the best choice, trying to avoid the sauces which often incorporate oil or other fats. Don't have dessert if you are not hungry, but if you do eat dessert, something fruit based (such as fruit salad) or meringue, will be healthier than cake or pastries.

A definite "red flag" to anyone with a weight problem is pastry (apart from filo pastry). Puff pastry is particularly calorific. It seems common for TV chefs to extol the virtues of ready-made puff pastry but I am of an age when girls were all taught cookery at school (the boys had to do woodwork). Anyone who has ever made puff pastry will recall it is an exercise in trying to incorporate as much butter as is physically possible into a flour mix. Don't eat pies at all, unless they are made from filo pastry, which has little fat. If you particularly like pies, it is sometimes possible to make a substitute using pizza dough instead of pastry, which does not taste quite the same but gives an acceptable result.

How to get this healthy food to become your normal regime? Of course, the individual is best placed to see how this can work for them. A different approach will be needed depending on lifestyle, occupation and cultural preferences, so the following suggestions may be helpful or not:

- *Eat breakfast* even if it is just toast and marmalade. Cereals, milk and fruit have been found to be a particularly good combination when weight is an issue. If you can, choose the wholegrain cereals. If you particularly like an English breakfast, then construct one with food such as grilled bacon with the fat removed, boiled/poached egg, grilled mushrooms and tomatoes. Toast is fine but don't make fried bread and avoid sausages.

- *Lunch* might be taken at work and this can present a problem if you are not in control of the available food as you would be at home. One way of having control over what you eat is to make your own healthy sandwiches (such as ham, tuna, chicken, lean roast meat, salad etc) and if you work in an office where everyone tends to buy sandwiches anyway, this will not ruin your social life. However, if everyone eats at a canteen, you can't spend your life sat in the corner of the office with your own lunch as a solitary figure. Perhaps there is something in the canteen that resembles nutritious food - roast chicken, a baked potato, salad or plain vegetables? Some canteens serve predominately high fat, calorie dense foods, such as pies and deep fried chips. If there really is not anything suitable, perhaps you could take something to work to eat late morning (such as a bagel with ketchup and lean bacon) which would be quite filling. If you then join your colleagues in the canteen, you will not be hungry and can have a cup of coffee, or some fruit.

Soups can be good for lunch and they are surprisingly easy to make and quite filling. There are lots of soup recipes available online, just avoid those that add cream or use a lot of fat.

Fruit and yoghurt are suitable desserts - if you can, add your own fruit to plain yoghurt, rather than buying processed ready prepared fruit yoghurt.

- *Evening meals* for anyone with a weight problem can be based on any sort of lean meat, poultry or fish cooked without fat. Boiled or baked vegetables are also fine. Pasta can be used - it is easier to portion if you weigh it before cooking. Most people find around 80g of dried pasta per person is about right. You can make oven potato wedges with just a small amount of oil, but if you have to use pre-prepared oven chips, there are some available that are made with just sunflower oil and potato and they contain less than 5% fat. It is a good idea to weigh out the portion size as directed on the packet before cooking the chips.

Constructing the sort of food you normally like to eat, in a way that contains less fat and is healthier, is more likely to be successful than forcing yourself to eat food that you don't like or enjoy. For instance, if your family like Spaghetti Bolognese, this can be made in a healthy fashion. Weigh the pasta and use either extra lean mince or dry-fry the mince first, then put it into a sieve so that the fat drains off, before incorporating it into the sauce. Using the smallest amount of oil possible to make the sauce and omitting the parmesan cheese makes the meal less calorie dense. You could add a salad, and if you put bread on the table, don't put butter or oil with it.

If you often order take away pizza or eat frozen pizza then making your own is not difficult and can be healthier and much cheaper than having it delivered (recipe suggestions are at the end of this chapter).

If you like Mexican food, just adapt the recipes so that the fat content is much reduced. Nigella Lawson has a good recipe for corn breaded topped chilli in her book *Feast,* and I have suggested ways in which you could lower the fat content at the end of this chapter.

- ***Snacks and desserts.*** If you tend to eat between meals, then having a snack food available which is naturally low in fat and healthy, means that you will be less likely to snack on the only snack food that is commercially available, which tends to be much less healthy. Any type of fruit makes a healthy snack but it is not very filling. Even eating toast and jam will be better than eating, for instance, chocolate biscuits from a packet. Similarly, English muffins (not the cake type), crumpets, teacakes and malt loaf are all at the lower end of the calorie spectrum, as long as you stick to jams and don't put butter all over them. If you need cake, a tea loaf is made without fat. It can be sliced and the slices individually frozen. You can then take a piece out of the freezer when you need it and leave it to defrost. This has a similar consistency and appearance to fruit cake - there is no need to put butter on it. There are recipes online, or Nigella Lawson's book *Feast* has a recipe for "fruit tea loaf".

Scones are easy to make, low in fat and can be frozen. Fresh fruit is one of the better desserts; you can eat it with yoghurt or made into fruit salad. Other desserts that are lower in calories include stewed fruit, baked apples, custard and meringues with a small amount of Greek yoghurt and fruit. A meringue with a little Greek yoghurt, covered in peaches and raspberries and a small amount of maple syrup, might give you something that looked a bit more like a traditional dessert.

- *Birthdays, Christmas and Celebrations* can be a particularly difficult time if you have a weight problem. It is a good idea to reduce the amount of high fat food that is available in your household. It might also be helpful to mention to anyone likely to give you a gift, that you are trying to lose weight, and are hoping not to receive chocolates or confectionary this year. If you do end up with boxes of chocolates, it might be better to re-wrap them and pass them on to someone else.

Birthdays are traditionally marked with a cake and something based on meringue, fruit and yoghurt might do as a substitute. Alternatively, you could make a whisked sponge cake, which has very little fat compared to traditional cake.

At Christmas, making sure you have a supply of pleasant food that is naturally low in fat, and avoiding the purchase of the kind of snack food that is widely available and often incorporates puff pastry, will help. Buy lots of fruit and avoid the sausage rolls and vol-au-vents. Christmas dinner is not too calorific if the skin is removed before eating the turkey, the vegetables are boiled or baked rather than roasted, and the stuffing is bread based (such as sage and onion) rather than containing sausage meat. Avoid the sausages and rolled bacon that sometimes accompany the meal. Christmas pudding is often fairly low in fat (if you buy it, the fat content will be on the packet) as is custard, but avoid brandy butter. Avoid mince pies at all cost, unless they are made with filo pastry. It is the pastry that is the problem generally, not the mincemeat. As we have already mentioned, if you have a weight problem, it is better to try and stick to your normal healthy eating plan over Christmas as much as you can.

What about alcohol?

It is worth considering alcohol intake, because if your alcohol intake is high, this could be contributing a lot of calories to your diet, with little nutritional benefit. For instance, wine contains about 125 calories per 175ml glass (small glass). A pint (570mls) of lager or ale is around 250 calories, and a gin or vodka and tonic is 126 calories. If drinking is part of your social life, you will not wish to cut it out altogether, but if you stick to the government's recommended maximum daily intake or less, you will not be consuming too many extra calories. For men, this limit is 3 or 4 units of alcohol per day, which is the equivalent of a pint and a half of 4% beer. For women, it is 2 or 3 units a day, which is one (175ml/6fl oz) glass of wine. If you are going over these values by any significant amount there is a risk to health as well as weight.

You can cut down the amount of alcohol by switching to smaller bottles of beer rather than pints, or announcing in the pub that you are switching to half pints, rather than pints, if pub drinking is part of your social life. I know that there is an absurd "macho" thing about men drinking pints in the UK, but if you are too shy to switch to halves because you are worried about what other people think, then you really are not very brave at all.

Drinking spritzers (white wine with carbonated water) is one way of diluting the alcohol. Certainly, the health limit of one glass of wine for women, some would find quite low, and this dilution might help. There are some nice sparkling mineral waters available now which are calorie free, and some soft fruit based drinks have been packaged into fancy bottles which may make you feel less deprived in the pub.

What about the budget?

It has been shown to be more expensive to have a diet of healthy fresh food than a diet of high fat, energy dense, processed food. It is going to be much easier to eat healthy food if you are wealthy. However, in the present economic climate many of us are managing on a reduced income and food is already a large proportion of our disposable income. Planning meals in advance and taking advantage of special offers on healthy foods can help with budgeting, as can buying seasonal foods and eating more vegetables than fruit, as fruit tends to cost more. It is probably easier to shop online, where prices are better displayed and comparisons made for you (sorting by "lowest price first") compared to standing in a supermarket, trying to work out the cost per kg/lb yourself.

If you have even a small garden, planting an apple or plum tree (which grow well in the UK) can give you a lot of free food in a year when the weather is reasonable. You get the added bonus of the blossom in the spring - apple blossom is very pretty. If you are having an apple tree, it might also be worth planting a blackberry plant. Blackberries are easy to grow and freeze well if you have a surplus. I am not sure how economic it is to grow many other foods. If you are a good gardener or have an allotment, I expect you have worked out how to do it, but I tend to find that the crops of vegetables are nothing like the picture on the seed packet. By the time you've bought the seeds and other items such as compost, it is debatable whether it saves any money. Some things do seem easier to grow - runner beans can give large crops. Rosemary grows quite well in the UK, as do mint and thyme. If you can have a few plants it is much cheaper than buying fresh herbs from the supermarket. Ask at the local garden centre for advice about which plants grow well and produce heavy crops, in your area.

The other resource that you might consider when planning changes to your diet, is a cookery book that suggests ways of making healthy, low fat food, that tastes good. For many of us, it will also be important that the food does not take too long to prepare and is of low cost. Despite there being plenty of cookery books available, very few fit these criteria. Many of the "celebrity chefs" seem to have no concept of a family budget, are too free with the fat and oil in their cooking, and produce dishes that require multiple stages of production, a long time to prepare and mountains of washing-up.

The chef Jamie Oliver notably tried to tackle poor diet in the North of England, in his television programmes. Whilst his aims were good, he obviously has little idea what a normal family budget looks like. Expecting people on very low income to buy salmon and coriander is absurd. His food is certainly very good and tastes delicious. However, I have been given a copy of his *Fifteen Minute Meals* and it took me an hour and a quarter to make the meal - and the cost was considerably higher than we normally spend. It would be helpful if he could find out what a normal family's budget for food was, and then plan a week's meals to fit this budget, starting from a household with just a few items in the fridge and not the normal extensive range of herbs, spices, flavoured oil and so forth that he is accustomed to having available.

Since I wrote the above paragraph, Jamie Oliver has brought out a TV series of "budget meals". So far, I have only seen one programme, but he started by cooking a shoulder of pork which he then used to make more meals, using a variety of bottled sauces. The pork alone cost £28 ($46), so his idea of budget cooking seems to be "budgeting for the wealthy." Anyone who is really short of money could not contemplate spending this amount. If you are out of work in the U.K. the "job seeker benefit" is £67 ($111) a week. I'd like him to try a little harder and work out how to make healthy, delicious meals with the sort of money that many families have at their disposal. If he can write a book that tells you how to make delicious healthy food for a family for a week, on an average budget, only using what he buys at a regular supermarket with no stock cupboard - then that would definitely be worth buying.

I cannot recommend any one cookery book but thinking what you would like to eat and then looking on Google for a healthy way of making it, is quite a good option (and it is also free). For instance, if you like to eat chicken curry, putting "healthy low fat recipe for chicken curry" into Google, will come up with several choices that should meet your needs. Just putting "healthy low fat recipe for ...." before your dish, usually produces a good result.

If your budget is not too stretched, try and get a dishwasher. If you are doing more home cooking and are time limited, it is virtually an essential, as it keeps the kitchen much tidier and cuts down the amount of time spent in the kitchen considerably. It doesn't have to be an expensive dishwasher - they do not seem to differ much in design.

Changing attitude to food

You might, by now, have identified some of you own attitudes to food that are contributing to a weight problem. Your plan might consider ways in which a tendency to eat in a manner which is emotional, uncontrolled, or too restrained, can be changed. You might also need to work on a tendency to apply dichotomous thinking to food issues, which has also been shown to be unhelpful. If you have a family, they too might benefit from a normalisation of the way in which food issues are considered. If you can avoid referring to food as "good" or "bad" in front of children, this will help them to have a more normal view of food, as they often mimic adult attitudes. In the supermarket, "look at those shiny red apples, I expect they are delicious", or "those tomatoes are really ripe and smell nice", are probably better comments for a child to hear than, "I suppose we'd better buy some vegetables and if we eat the broccoli, then we can have something nice like chocolate cake". If children view vegetables as an unattractive food, they are not going to choose to eat them of their own volition.

Have a look at your favourite food list. If it all comes into the healthy, low fat food category, this is fine. However, if you have a weight problem there might well be some foods topping the list that are more difficult to construct from healthier ingredients. If your favourite food is pizza, then it is relatively easy to make a healthy version. If it is lasagne, then make up the meat sauce to be of low fat, and making a white sauce using predominately milk and flour is possible. This will reduce the fat content of the finished dish (directions towards specific recipes are listed at the end of this chapter). You see where we are going with this - deciding what you like to eat, and then making a version that is lower in fat, is generally possible.

However, what if your favourite food is something like chocolate? If you are not keen on chocolate, then omitting it from the diet will be quite possible, but for many people chocolate is one of their favourite food items. For a diet to be sustainable long term, it needs to include some of your favourites. There are various strategies you might consider to cope with the chocolate problem. It is in any case better to eat a small amount of decent quality chocolate, rather than a large amount of the chocolate which is commercially widely available but only contains a small proportion of cocoa bean.

You might try buying something like a 100g (3.5oz) bar of 70% cocoa dark chocolate, dividing it into squares, re-wrapping them individually in foil and then putting them out of sight in a non-transparent container, limiting yourself to one square a day. If you cannot manage this and are still likely to eat a whole week's chocolate in one day, then you need something else that will work for you. Perhaps buy one chocolate a day, or get someone else to keep them for you. In the worst case and if all else fails you could try some "do-it-yourself" aversion therapy. If your least favourite foods are, for instance, stilton and marmite, then every time you think of chocolate try and imagine it smeared in marmite on a slice of stilton. I would not recommend this though unless you are having real difficulties limiting one particular high fat food, as food should be enjoyable.

Chocolate is often a problem. I did hear of one woman whose husband worked as a buyer of chocolate and confectionary for a prestigious London store. He was given a lot of samples and despite her pleas not to bring them home, as she was concerned about her weight, these high quality chocolates would still find their way into the house. In the end, she would have to tip the chocolates out of the boxes into the baby's dirty nappy bin. She actually had to open up the old nappy sacks and tip the chocolates into them, as that way she was absolutely sure that she would not eat them.

Exercise and movement

Hopefully the chapter on exercise will have given you some idea of the extent to which exercise will help you to lose weight. Decide what exercise you need, taking into account your age, gender, weight and state of health. Your family doctor should check that what you have chosen is reasonable, and will not have a negative impact on your health. If you are not inclined to sport, walking seems to be the best form of exercise and most helpful in preventing weight regain. It doesn't have to be long distance fell walking, just an extra mile a day will make a big difference over time, but you need to tailor what you do to your own circumstances. If you are at the bigger end of the weight scale, walking might be the best exercise, or if there are problems with joints, perhaps try some gentle swimming. Incorporating some extra walking into your daily routine is probably going to make the most difference long term. If you can make this an enjoyable excursion, it is likely to be more sustainable than choosing something like tap dancing or hang-gliding. On the other hand, particularly if you are a young fit man, joining a gym and asking their advisors for a specific exercise regime tailored to your needs might be useful, if this appeals to you. Have another look at the chapter on exercise if you need more help deciding what to do.

Social support

If you have a supportive spouse or family, then enlisting their support to help with your new strategy for eating and exercise will be advantageous. If you have a family, then having a kitchen stocked with plenty of healthy food, good bread, pasta, pulses, lean meat, poultry, fish, eggs, fruit and vegetables etc will be to their benefit too. There is no absolute need to buy cakes, biscuits, crisps, sweets or pies - no one ever died from a deficiency of these items. Hopefully, you can get the family on board and point out that although you are all going to have to do a little more cooking and food preparation, the end results should taste much better.

If you live alone or have an unsupportive family, then maybe you can look to a friend for help. You could also consider joining one of the weight loss groups that hold meetings regularly. If you are thinking of this option, be careful what you join. I would be more concerned about groups that are heavily marketing their own diet products in the sessions. Also, how good a group is can depend on the quality of the group leader. A badly directed group, for instance, can concentrate on discussing who has eaten the most, or put on the most weight and be quite negative and unsupportive of those who have lost or maintained their weight. A supportive group would spend more time looking at strategies that people have found helpful to get to a healthy weight. It might also discuss ways of coping with the discrimination that larger people can encounter, particularly when they start to take exercise.

Monitoring weight and avoiding relapse

It does seem that regular weighing can be helpful, particularly when you have lost weight and need to avoid putting it back on. I would suggest that you monitor your weight at least once a week if you have, or have had, a significant weight problem. Take action early to correct it, if it goes up by as much as 3lbs (1.4kg), and you are more likely to be successful.

If you have a relapse, try not to think that all is lost and you might as well go back to the old ways. This is the type of thinking that is associated with weight regain. Instead, think something like, "I've put 5lbs (2.3kg) back on, but I had lost 3 stone (19kg). It is disappointing, but if I tackle this now I can get the 5lb (2.3kg) back off. I've already done it once. It's just a blip and I can get over this."

If the weight starts to go up, go back to looking at what you are eating, examine your bills, look in the fridge, have you kept up with the walking? Go back to what worked for you before, until you feel you are once again eating healthy food and have a reasonable level of activity.

Coping with the stigma of weight problems

This might be something you need to incorporate into your plan. You are more likely to encounter problems with weight discrimination if you are female, and if your excess weight is at the heavier end of the spectrum. What problems have you encountered and what do you think you could do to minimise them? I hope that the earlier chapters will have given you some ideas about what might work for you.

For instance, if you are large and want to join a gym, why not ring them up first? If you have an assertive personality you might want to be quite blunt on the phone and say something like, "I'm thinking of joining a gym. I am quite large, around 20 stone (127kg/280lbs). I want to know if you have a trainer that would be able to advise me about the best exercises for my size. Do you have equipment that would be suitable for someone of my size?" In this way, you will know what to expect when you get to the gym, and they are more likely to be organised to meet your needs, reducing the need for embarrassing discussions at the front desk.

You could also ask them about the sort of clothes that would be suitable to wear. You want to feel comfortable and unless you are really confident, probably not too exposed. Lycra is not compulsory. If you are less confident, you could always email or write to the gym and find out how helpful they would be. You are paying them for a service, so you have the right to ask questions. A good organisation will try to meet the needs of all its customers.

An individual approach to weight

Those people most successful at losing weight, and keeping it off, have found ways of adjusting their lifestyle and diet that suit them personally. I hope, by now, you will have found information in this book that will help you to formulate some changes that will be helpful. Do check with your family doctor first that any changes that you are going to make will suit you, and are appropriate for your state of health - then monitor your weight regularly to check that your plan is working. The first aim is to stop putting weight on, then to gradually and slowly reduce weight, until you get to a weight which is more acceptable to yourself and nearer to the healthy weight band. Weight loss, to be sustainable, should not be too rapid. Whilst you can discuss the amount of weight and rate of loss with your doctor, in general, one or two pounds loss each week is quite enough. Keep the plan under review and make changes if it is not working for you. Not putting any more weight on, is a success in itself and a good starting point.

Remember that being overweight is not your fault. It is something that will happen to those with the genetic predisposition to add weight, that are living in modern society, with a wide availability of high fat processed foods. Your slimmer friends and colleagues do not have more willpower than you, or any greater moral fibre. They just don't have the genes to put on weight designed to help survive famine conditions. It is reasonable to be assertive in your need for help with this problem, whether at the doctors, the gym, at work or in any other social situation. The increase in the proportion of people who have an excess weight problem over the last few decades is not irreversible, and focusing on healthy eating and lifestyle will help to reverse this trend.

The website address that will be associated with this book is:

www.theweightissue.com

Appendix

Recipes mentioned in Chapter 7

Using Google can be very helpful - put your favourite meals into the search engine prefaced by "healthy low fat recipe for." For example, if you particularly like beef burgers, putting "healthy low fat recipe for beef burgers" into Google will produce many suitable recipes including:

http://www.bbcgoodfood.com/recipes/3413/beef-and-salsa-burgers - a beef burger recipe based on using extra lean mince (which can now be purchased with only 5% fat content from some major supermarkets).

Soup

Soups can be good for lunch and are surprisingly easy to make and quite filling. The key for a healthy soup is to use the minimum of oil or butter to fry the chopped vegetables and onion for a few minutes (less than a teaspoon of oil or butter is often enough). Then add the stock (an organic stock cube is fine, or homemade stock if you skim all the fat off first). Simmer until the vegetables are cooked through and blend or liquidise and season. There are lots of soup recipes available online, just avoid those that add cream or use a large amount of fat.

Pizza

Ingredients:

- 325ml lukewarm water
- 1/2 teaspoon sugar
- 7g dried yeast (NOT easybake yeast)
- 500g strong white bread flour (make sure the packet says "strong")
- 1/2 tablespoon salt

- passata (around 4 or 5 tablespoons)
- chilli flakes or oregano (optional)
- low fat toppings - such as lean bacon, ham or chicken, chopped or thinly sliced peppers, mushrooms, onions, tomatoes, tinned sweetcorn, pineapple - most of the vegetable toppings that you would normally have. (Avoid sausage, pepperoni or much cheese - although you might need a very small amount of mozzarella to scatter over the top, in order to get the other toppings to stick.)

If you often order take-away pizza, or eat frozen pizza then making your own is not difficult and can be healthier and much cheaper than having it delivered. Just put 325ml of lukewarm water into a jug and add half a teaspoon of sugar and 7g of ordinary dried yeast (about 7 mls or just under 1 1/2 teaspoons - NOT "easy bake" yeast - Allinsons do yeast in a yellow tin which is fine).

Put 500g of strong white bread making flour into a bowl, make a well in the centre and sprinkle half a tablespoon of salt around the outer edge of the flour. When the yeast mixture has started to froth on top, pour it into the centre of the bowl and mix all together with a wooden spoon and then your hands. Depending on the flour, you might need another tablespoon of water to draw the mixture together. Knead the dough on the table for 2-3 minutes using the minimum of extra flour to dust the table first. Then cover loosely with cling film and leave for 15 minutes. Re-knead for a minute (you will need to sprinkle a little flour on the table first) then cut the dough into 3 or 4 pieces depending whether you want a small or medium pizza. Roll each piece out to the thickness you want depending whether you like a thin or thick base (a 25cm diameter circle or a smaller rectangle). Put each piece onto an oiled baking tray. If you only have a couple of trays and two racks in your oven, put some of the pizzas on oiled foil sheets so that you can lift them onto the trays and cook as a second batch on the foil. Preheat the oven to 230 degrees C (446F).

The pizza bases need to rest for 30 minutes before you put them in the oven but you can start putting the toppings on during this time. Passata can be used as a tomato sauce unless you particularly want to make your own sauce. Use it as it is, or add a few chilli flakes if you like spice, then put 1-2 tablespoons onto each pizza and spread it out, leaving the edges free from sauce. Then put on whatever toppings you like, omitting most of the cheese or sausage type toppings for anyone with a weight problem.

Make sure that the toppings are dried with kitchen roll first, if necessary. If you put wet ingredients (such as tinned bits of pineapple or sweetcorn) on top, without drying it, the base might go soggy. Suitable toppings include ham, lean bits of grilled bacon, pineapple, thinly sliced peppers, courgette (zucchini), onions, sliced mushroom, sliced chillies, sliced tomatoes (remove seeds), anchovies (wipe off the oil first) and oregano. If you find the absence of mozzarella difficult, just tear up a small amount of mozzarella, dot it across the top and use the rest for the pizza of someone who does not have a weight problem. If you have children, they will enjoy adding their own pizza toppings. Cook the pizza in the hot oven for around 10-15 minutes depending on the size, so look at it after 10 minutes. It is cooked when the dough is starting to look golden brown around the edge and under the base.

To adapt a recipe for chilli

If you like Mexican food, just adapt the recipes so the fat content is much reduced. Nigella Lawson has a good recipe for corn breaded topped chilli in her book *Feast,* which she has also put online at:

http://www.nigella.com/recipes/view/cornbread-topped-chilli-con-carne-126

You can make it lower in fat by using extra lean mince (5% fat) or dry frying the mince first to melt the fat, which you can then drain off. You can also considerably reduce the amount of oil used to brown the onions at the start - perhaps from 4 to 1 tablespoon, as long as you stir and keep an eye on it. The cornbread as she suggests should be fine, you will need the oil here but it serves a lot of people. Don't worry about using buttermilk - despite its name it is not particularly high in fat.

If you have weight issues and are using this recipe you can omit the cheese which it suggests is sprinkled on top and also omit the sour cream and just have a little guacamole. Similarly, her subsequent recipe in the same book is for vegetarian chilli with cornbread topping (page 402) and this is also good, and a cheap way of feeding many people. If you similarly cut down on the amount of fat that is used at the start, the dish will be much less calorific but still taste good.

Scones

Ingredients:

- 500g self-raising flour
- 1/2 teaspoon cream of tartar
- 70g butter
- 3 tablespoons caster sugar
- 100g dried fruit such as sultanas (optional)
- 300mls milk

Scones are easy to make, low in fat and can be frozen. To make scones, pre-heat an oven to 220 degrees C (428F) and mix 500g of self-raising flour with half a teaspoon of cream of tartar. Rub in 70g of butter and then stir in three tablespoons of caster sugar. If you want, you can then stir in 100g of dried fruit, such as sultanas. Mix in the milk to form a dough (add around 250mls first and then the rest if you need it - flours tend to vary and the dough should not be wet).

Roll out on a lightly floured surface, making sure you don't go too thin - the scones should be at least 2.5cm thick. Cut out using a 5cm cutter to make around 15 scones and put onto lightly oiled metal baking trays. Brush only the tops with beaten egg and bake for about 10 minutes. They might need another 2 or 3 minutes depending on your oven. They should be risen and brown on top and on the base. Put on a wire rack to cool and serve cut in half with jam (no butter or cream). If you make a batch and you want to eat them from the freezer, just put them on a tray in a cold oven and turn the temperature up to 200 degrees C (392F) and heat for around 15 minutes until hot all the way through (cut one in half to check, as ovens vary). Alternatively, just leave them out of the freezer for a few hours to defrost.

Sponge cake

Ingredients:

- 4 eggs
- 100g plain flour
- 1/2 teaspoon baking powder
- 100g caster sugar
- jam or conserve for filling

To make a whisked sponge; oil and line two 18cm circular cake tins and preheat the oven to 180 degrees C (356F). Separate four eggs and put the yolks in one bowl and the whites in another. Sieve 100g plain flour and 1/2 teaspoon baking powder into a third bowl. Whisk the egg whites until they form stiff peaks, starting slowly and gradually increasing the speed. Then whisk together the egg yolks with 100g of caster sugar, again starting off slowly and gradually increasing the speed, for several minutes, until the mixture has gone pale and increased in volume.

You then use a large metal spoon to gently fold the egg white alternately with some of the flour into the yolk mixture - use alternate egg white and flour, starting and finishing with the egg white. If you use about a quarter of the egg white and a third of the flour each time, this should work out correctly. Be gentle so as not to lose the air bubbles, but also do not take too long. Divide the mixture between the cake tins and cook in the centre of the oven for 20-25 minutes, and then check if the cake is cooked. The sponges are cooked when they are light brown, well risen and spring back when touched. Cool in the tin for one minute, then tip out onto greaseproof paper that has been sprinkled with caster sugar. Then cool the sponges on a wire rack and when completely cold, sandwich together with jam. A glace or fondant icing on top will have much less fat than a butter cream icing. This cake is best eaten the day it is made and does not keep as long as a cake which incorporates butter.

Mince Pies with Filo pastry

Ingredients:

- one packet of filo pastry
- one jar of mincemeat
- sunflower oil to oil the tins
- melted butter
- icing sugar to dust (optional)

To make mince pies with filo pastry, cut the filo into squares slightly bigger than the depressions in the metal baking sheet you are using for mince pie making. Lightly oil the tins. For each pie, put in 3 or 4 squares on top of each other at an angle to one another, lightly brushing each layer with melted butter (use the minimum) so that they adhere to one another. Put a large teaspoonful of mincemeat into the middle of each pie and cook in a hot oven (200C/400F) for about 10-15 minutes, until golden. Cool on a wire rack before eating. If you wish, you can dust with icing sugar before serving. These pies are best eaten on the day they are made, as filo pastry does not keep as well as pastry with a higher proportion of fat.

Lasagne

If you like lasagne, you can adapt the standard recipe by making up the meat sauce using the minimum of oil and lean mince, or draining off the fat first after dry frying standard mince. Make a white sauce by whisking up cold milk and some flour - for instance as described by Delia Smith online at http://www.deliaonline.com/recipes/type-of-dish/sauce/fatless-white-sauce.html
Getting the cheese flavour to the sauce without adding a lot of calories is more difficult, but can be done by adding a spoonful of naturally low fat cream cheese.

References

Chapter 1 References

Stunkard, Albert J., et al. "An adoption study of human obesity." New England Journal of Medicine 314.4 (1986): 193-198.

Shalikashvili J and Shelton H, "The latest national security threat: Obesity" Washington Post April 30th 2010.

Allison, D. B., et al. "The heritability of body mass index among an international sample of monozygotic twins reared apart." International journal of obesity 20 (1996): 501-506.

Bouchard, Claude, et al. "The response to long-term overfeeding in identical twins." New England Journal of Medicine 322.21 (1990): 1477-1482.

Friedman, Jeffrey M. "Obesity: Causes and control of excess body fat." Nature459.7245 (2009): 340-342.

Friedman, Jeffrey M. "A war on obesity, not the obese." Science 299.5608 (2003): 856-858.

Spiegelman, Bruce M., and Jeffrey S. Flier. "Obesity and the regulation review of energy balance." Cell 104 (2001): 531-543.

Kopelman, Peter G. "Obesity as a medical problem." NATURE-LONDON- (2000): 635-643.

Friedman, Jeffrey M. "Modern science versus the stigma of obesity." Nature medicine 10.6 (2004): 563-569.

Friedman, Jeffrey M. "Obesity in the new millennium." Nature 404.6778 (2000): 632-634.

Blundell, J. E. and Gillett, A. (2001), Control of Food Intake in the Obese. Obesity Research, 9: 263S–270S. doi: 10.1038/oby.2001.129

Farooqi, I. Sadaf, et al. "Beneficial effects of leptin on obesity, T cell hyporesponsiveness, and neuroendocrine/metabolic dysfunction of human congenital leptin deficiency." Journal of Clinical Investigation 110.8 (2002): 1093-1104.

Havel, Peter J., et al. "High-fat meals reduce 24-h circulating leptin concentrations in women." Diabetes 48.2 (1999): 334-341.

Tsigos, Constantine, et al. "Management of obesity in adults: European clinical practice guidelines." Obesity facts 1.2 (2008): 106-116.

Michaelowa, Axel, and Björn Dransfeld. "Greenhouse gas benefits of fighting obesity." Ecological Economics 66.2 (2008): 298-308.

Pereira, Mark A., et al. "Fast-food habits, weight gain, and insulin resistance (the CARDIA study): 15-year prospective analysis." The Lancet 365.9453 (2005): 36-42.

Young, Lisa R., and Marion Nestle. "The contribution of expanding portion sizes to the US obesity epidemic." Journal Information 92.2 (2002).

Van Ittersum, Koert, and Brian Wansink. "Plate size and color suggestibility: The Delboeuf Illusion's bias on serving and eating behavior." Journal of Consumer Research, Forthcoming (2011).

Rolls, Barbara J., Erin L. Morris, and Liane S. Roe. "Portion size of food affects energy intake in normal-weight and overweight men and women." The American journal of clinical nutrition 76.6 (2002): 1207-1213.

Levitsky, David A., and Trisha Youn. "The more food young adults are served, the more they overeat." The Journal of nutrition 134.10 (2004): 2546-2549.

Rolls, Barbara J., et al. "Increasing the portion size of a packaged snack increases energy intake in men and women." Appetite 42.1 (2004): 63-69.

Wansink, Brian. "Can package size accelerate usage volume?" The Journal of Marketing (1996): 1-14.

Wansink, Brian, Koert Van Ittersum, and James E. Painter. "How descriptive food names bias sensory perceptions in restaurants." Food Quality and Preference 16.5 (2005): 393-400.

Wansink, Brian. "Environmental Factors That Increase the Food Intake and Consumption Volume of Unknowing Consumers*." Annu. Rev. Nutr. 24 (2004): 455-479.

North, Adrian C., David J. Hargreaves, and Jennifer McKendrick. "In-store music affects product choice." Nature (1997).

Steinberg, Sandon A., and Richard F. Yalch. "When eating begets buying: the effects of food samples on obese and nonobese shoppers." Journal of Consumer Research (1978): 243-246.

Nisbett, Richard E., and David E. Kanouse. "Obesity, food deprivation, and supermarket shopping behavior." Journal of personality and social psychology 12.4 (1969): 289.

Chandon, Pierre, and Brian Wansink. "When are stockpiled products consumed faster? A convenience-salience framework of postpurchase consumption incidence and quantity." Journal of Marketing Research (2002): 321-335.

Lewin, Alexandra, Lauren Lindstrom, and Marion Nestle. "Commentary: Food Industry Promises to Address Childhood Obesity: Preliminary Evaluation."Journal of Public Health Policy (2006): 327-348.

Gross, Lee S., et al. "Increased consumption of refined carbohydrates and the epidemic of type 2 diabetes in the United States: an ecologic assessment."The American journal of clinical nutrition 79.5 (2004): 774-779.

Forshee, Richard A., et al. "A critical examination of the evidence relating high fructose corn syrup and weight gain." Critical reviews in food science and nutrition 47.6 (2007): 561-582.

Prentice, Andrew M., and Susan A. Jebb. "Obesity in Britain: gluttony or sloth?." BMJ: British Medical Journal 311.7002 (1995): 437.

Mozaffarian, Dariush, et al. "Changes in diet and lifestyle and long-term weight gain in women and men." New England Journal of Medicine 364.25 (2011): 2392-2404.

Kopelman, Peter G. "Obesity as a medical problem." NATURE-LONDON-

(2000): 635-643.

Gore, Stacy A., et al. "Television viewing and snacking." Eating behaviors 4.4 (2003): 399-405.

Rissanen, A. M., et al. "Determinants of weight gain and overweight in adult Finns." European journal of clinical nutrition 45.9 (1991): 419.

Smith, Trenton G., Christiana Stoddard, and Michael G. Barnes. "Why the poor get fat: Weight gain and economic insecurity." Forum for Health Economics & Policy. Vol. 12. No. 2. Berkeley Electronic Press, 2009.

Dubé, Laurette, Jordan L. LeBel, and Ji Lu. "Affect asymmetry and comfort food consumption." Physiology & Behavior 86.4 (2005): 559-567.

Rozin, Paul, et al. "The Ecology of Eating Smaller Portion Sizes in France Than in the United States Help Explain the French Paradox." Psychological Science14.5 (2003): 450-454.

Wansink, Brian, Collin R. Payne, and Pierre Chandon. "Internal and external cues of meal cessation: The French paradox redux?." Obesity (2007).

Oliver, Georgina, Jane Wardle, and E. Leigh Gibson. "Stress and food choice: a laboratory study." Psychosomatic medicine 62.6 (2000): 853-865.

Drewnowski, Adam, et al. "Food preferences in human obesity: carbohydrates versus fats." Appetite 18.3 (1992): 207-221.

Markus C R Effects of carbohydrates on brain tryptophan availability and stress performance, Biological Psychology. Volume 76, Issues 1-2 September 2007 pages 83-90

Macht, Michael, and Jochen Mueller. "Immediate effects of chocolate on experimentally inducedmood states." Appetite 49.3 (2007): 667-674.

Leigh Gibson, Edward. "Emotional influences on food choice: sensory, physiological and psychological pathways." Physiology & behavior 89.1 (2006): 53-61.

Christakis, Nicholas A., and James H. Fowler. "The spread of obesity in a large social network over 32 years." New England journal of medicine 357.4 (2007): 370-379.

Clive Thompson Are your Frieds Making You Fat? New York Times September 13 2009

Wansink, Brian. "Environmental factors that unknowingly increase a consumer's food intake and consumption volume." Annual Review of Nutrition24 (2004): 455-479.

Salvy, Sarah-Jeanne, Elizabeth Kieffer, and Leonard H. Epstein. "Effects of social context on overweight and normal-weight children's food selection."Eating behaviors 9.2 (2008): 190-196.

Salvy, Sarah-Jeanne, et al. "The presence of friends increases food intake in youth." The American journal of clinical nutrition 90.2 (2009): 282-287.

de Luca, Rayleen V., and Manly N. Spigelman. "Effects of models on food intake of obese and non-obese female college students." Canadian Journal of Behavioural Science/Revue canadienne des sciences du comportement 11.2 (1979): 124.

Young, Meredith E., et al. "Food for thought. What you eat depends on your sex and eating companions." Appetite 53.2 (2009): 268-271.

Salvy, Sarah-Jeanne, et al. "Effects of social influence on eating in couples, friends and strangers." Appetite 49.1 (2007): 92-99.

Vartanian, Lenny R., C. Peter Herman, and Janet Polivy. "Consumption stereotypes and impression management: How you are what you eat." Appetite48.3 (2007): 265-277.7

Herman, C. Peter, Deborah A. Roth, and Janet Polivy. "Effects of the presence of others on food intake: a normative interpretation." Psychological Bulletin129.6 (2003): 873.

Lee, Alan B., and Morton Goldman. "Effect of staring on normal and overweight students." The Journal of Social Psychology 108.2 (1979): 165-169.

Salvy, Sarah-Jeanne, et al. "The role of familiarity on modeling of eating and food consumption in children." Appetite 50.2 (2008): 514-518.

Davis, Esa M., et al. "Racial, ethnic, and socioeconomic differences in the incidence of obesity related to childbirth." American Journal of Public Health99.2 (2009): 294.

Sobal, Jeffrey, Barbara S. Rauschenbach, and Edward A. Frongillo. "Marital status, fatness and obesity." Social Science & Medicine 35.7 (1992): 915-923.

Brunner, Eric J., Tarani Chandola, and Michael G. Marmot. "Prospective effect of job strain on general and central obesity in the Whitehall II Study." American journal of epidemiology 165.7 (2007): 828-837.

Wansink, Brian, James E. Painter, and Jill North. "Bottomless Bowls: Why Visual Cues of Portion Size May Influence Intake* &ast." Obesity 13.1 (2005): 93-100.

Vartanian, Lenny R., C. Peter Herman, and Brian Wansink. "Are we aware of the external factors that influence our food intake?." Health Psychology 27.5 (2008): 533.

Caldwell, Clare, and Sally A. Hibbert. "The influence of music tempo and musical preference on restaurant patrons' behavior." Psychology and Marketing19.11 (2002): 895-917.

Wansink, Brian, Koert van Ittersum, and James E. Painter. "How descriptive food names bias sensory perceptions in restaurants." Food Quality and Preference 16.5 (2005): 393-400.

Wansink, Brian. "Environmental factors that unknowingly increase a consumer's food intake and consumption volume." Annual Review of Nutrition24 (2004): 455-479.

North, Adrian C., David J. Hargreaves, and Jennifer McKendrick. "In-store music affects product choice." Nature; Nature (1997).

Meiselman, Herbert L., et al. "Effect of effort on meal selection and meal acceptability in a student cafeteria." Appetite 23.1 (1994): 43-56.

Rozin, Paul, et al. "Nudge to nobesity I: Minor changes in accessibility decrease food intake." Judgment and Decision Making 6.4 (2011): 323-332.

Herman, C. Peter, Marion P. Olmsted, and Janet Polivy. "Obesity, externality, and susceptibility to social influence: An integrated analysis." Journal of Personality and Social Psychology 45.4 (1983): 926.

Wansink, Brian, James E. Painter, and Yeon-Kyung Lee. "The office candy dish: proximity's influence on estimated and actual consumption." International journal of obesity 30.5 (2006): 871-875.

Rodin, Judith. "Effects of distraction on performance of obese and normal subjects." Journal of Comparative and Physiological Psychology 83.1 (1973): 68.

Rolls, Barbara J., et al. "Sensory specific satiety in man." Physiology & Behavior 27.1 (1981): 137-142.

Iyengar, Sheena S., and Mark R. Lepper. "When choice is demotivating: Can one desire too much of a good thing?." Journal of personality and social psychology 79.6 (2000): 995.

Steinberg, Sandon A., and Richard F. Yalch. "When eating begets buying: the effects of food samples on obese and nonobese shoppers." Journal of Consumer Research (1978): 243-246.

Nisbett, Richard E., and David E. Kanouse. "Obesity, food deprivation, and supermarket shopping behavior." Journal of personality and social psychology12.4 (1969): 289.

Wansink, B., J. E. Painter, and K. Van Ittersum. "Bowl-size, spoon-size, and consumption intake at the ice cream social." Under review (2004). IAL 2004 WANSINK ET AL.

Wansink, Brian, Koert Van Ittersum, and James E. Painter. "Ice cream illusions: bowls, spoons, and self-served portion sizes." American journal of preventive medicine 31.3 (2006): 240-243.

Rolls, Barbara J., Elizabeth A. Bell, and Bethany A. Waugh. "Increasing the volume of a food by incorporating air affects satiety in men." The American journal of clinical nutrition 72.2 (2000): 361-368.

Cohen, Deborah, and Thomas A. Farley. "Peer Reviewed: Eating as an Automatic Behavior." Preventing chronic disease 5.1 (2008).

Baumeister, Roy F., et al. "Ego depletion: is the active self a limited resource?." Journal of personality and social psychology 74.5 (1998): 1252.

Kahn, Barbara E., and Brian Wansink. "The influence of assortment structure on perceived variety and consumption quantities." Journal of Consumer Research 30.4 (2004): 519-533.

Rasmussen, Mette, et al. "Determinants of fruit and vegetable consumption among children and adolescents: a review of the literature. Part I: quantitative studies." International Journal of Behavioral Nutrition and Physical Activity 3.1 (2006): 22.

Atkinson, Richard L. "Human adenovirus-36 and childhood obesity "International Journal of Pediatric Obesity 6.S1 (2011) : 2-6

Na, H. N., H. Kim, and J. H. Nam. "Novel genes and cellular pathways related to infection with adenovirus-36 as an obesity agent in human mesenchymal stem cells." International Journal of Obesity 36.2 (2011): 195-200.

Na, H. N., et al. "Association of human adenovirus-36 in overweight Korean adults." International Journal of Obesity (2011).

Friedman, Jeffrey M. "Obesity: Causes and control of excess body fat." Nature459.7245 (2009): 340-342.

Friedman, Jeffrey M. "Modern science versus the stigma of obesity." Nature medicine 10.6 (2004): 563-569.

Yanovski, Susan Z., and Jack A. Yanovski. "Obesity Prevalence in the United States—Up, Down, or Sideways?." New England Journal of Medicine 364.11 (2011): 987-989.

K. L., and S. A. Jebb. "Prevalence of obesity in Great Britain." Obesity reviews 6.1 (2005): 11-12. 2010.

Kopelman, Peter G. "Obesity as a medical problem." NATURE-LONDON-(2000): 635-643.

Gabbert, Charles, et al. "Adenovirus 36 and obesity in children and adolescents." Pediatrics 126.4 (2010): 721-726.

Consultation, W. H. O. "Obesity: preventing and managing the global epidemic." World Health Organization technical report series 894 (2000).

Prof. J. Friedman Rockefeller University Nature Medicine 10, 563 - 569 (2004) doi:10.1038/nm0604-563 Modern Science versus the stigma of obesity June 1 2004

Sobal, Jeffrey, Barbara S. Rauschenbach, and Edward A. Frongillo Jr. "Marital status, fatness and obesity." Social Science & Medicine 35.7 (1992): 915-923.

Chapter 2 References

Goldstein, David J. "Beneficial health effects of modest weight loss."International journal of obesity and related metabolic disorders: journal of the International Association for the Study of Obesity 16.6 (1992): 397.

Friedman, Jeffrey M. "Obesity in the new millennium." Nature 404.6778 (2000): 632-634.

Lew, EDWARD A. "Mortality and weight: insured lives and the American Cancer Society studies." Annals of internal medicine 103.6 (Pt 2) (1985): 1024.

Consultation, W. H. O. "Obesity: preventing and managing the global epidemic." World Health Organization technical report series 894 (2000).

Kopelman, Peter G. "Obesity as a medical problem." NATURE-LONDON-(2000): 635-643.

Manson, JoAnn E., et al. "Body weight and mortality among women." New England Journal of Medicine 333.11 (1995): 677-685.

Pörtner, Claus C., and Edwin S. Wong. "The Link between Parental and Offspring Longevity." (2013).

Mehta, Neil K., and Virginia W. Chang. "Mortality attributable to obesity among middle-aged adults in the United States." Demography 46.4 (2009): 851-872.

Narayan, KM Venkat, et al. "Lifetime risk for diabetes mellitus in the United States." JAMA: the journal of the American Medical Association 290.14 (2003): 1884-1890.

Sturm, Roland. "The effects of obesity, smoking, and drinking on medical problems and costs." Health Affairs 21.2 (2002): 245-253.

Thompson, David, et al. "Lifetime health and economic consequences of obesity." Archives of Internal Medicine 159.18 (1999): 2177.

Giovannucci, Edward, et al. "Obesity and benign prostatic hyperplasia."American journal of epidemiology 140.11 (1994): 989-1002.

Wang, Y. Claire, et al. "Health and economic burden of the projected obesity trends in the USA and the UK." The Lancet 378.9793 (2011): 815-825.

Stothard, Katherine J., et al. "Maternal overweight and obesity and the risk of congenital anomalies." JAMA: the journal of the American Medical Association301.6 (2009): 636-650.

Sheiner, Eyal, et al. "Maternal obesity as an independent risk factor for caesarean delivery." Paediatric and perinatal epidemiology 18.3 (2004): 196-201.

Calle, Eugenia E., and Rudolf Kaaks. "Overweight, obesity and cancer: epidemiological evidence and proposed mechanisms." Nature Reviews Cancer4.8 (2004): 579-591.

Stunkard, Albert J., and Thomas A. Wadden. "Psychological aspects of severe obesity." The American journal of clinical nutrition 55.2 (1992): 524S-532S.

Carpenter, Kenneth M., et al. "Relationships between obesity and DSM-IV major depressive disorder, suicide ideation, and suicide attempts: results from a general population study." American Journal of Public Health 90.2 (2000): 251.

Tsigos, Constantine, et al. "Management of obesity in adults: European clinical practice guidelines." Obesity facts 1.2 (2008): 106-116.

Rand, C. S., and A. M. Macgregor. "Successful weight loss following obesity surgery and the perceived liability of morbid obesity." International journal of obesity 15.9 (1991): 577.

Fairburn, Christopher G., and Kelly D. Brownell, eds. Eating disorders and obesity: A comprehensive handbook. Guilford Press, 2001.

Erlinger, Serge. "Gallstones in obesity and weight loss." European journal of gastroenterology & hepatology 12.12 (2000): 1347.

Jensen, Lars Bjørn, Flemming Quaade, and Ole Helmer Sørensen. "Bone loss accompanying voluntary weight loss in obese humans." Journal of Bone and Mineral Research 9.4 (1994): 459-463.

Wannamethee, S. Goya, A. Gerald Shaper, and Mary Walker. "Weight change, weight
fluctuation, and mortality." Ar Consultation, W. H. O. "Obesity: preventing and managing the global epidemic."

Consultation, W. H. O. "Obesity: preventing and managing the global epidemic." World Health Organization technical report series 894 (2000).

Duncan, Glen E. "The" fit but fat" concept revisited: population-based estimates using NHANES." International Journal of Behavioral Nutrition and Physical Activity 7.1 (2010): 1-5.

Blair, Steven N., and Suzanne Brodney. "Effects of physical inactivity and obesity on morbidity and mortality: current evidence and research issues."Medicine and science in sports and exercise 31 (1999): 646-662.

Blair, Steven N., and Tim S. Church. "The fitness, obesity, and health equation." JAMA: the journal of the American Medical Association 292.10 (2004): 1232-1234.

Blair, Steven N., Yiling Cheng, and J. Scott Holder. "Is physical activity or physical fitness more important in defining health benefits?." Medicine and Science in Sports and Exercise 33.6; SUPP (2001): 379-399.

Jane Brody, "Personal Health Fat but Fit; A myth about obesity is slowly being debunked," New York Times 2000/10/24

Reilly, J. J., et al. "Health consequences of obesity." Archives of disease in childhood 88.9 (2003): 748-752.

Gold, Diane R., et al. "Body-mass index as a predictor of incident asthma in prospective cohort of children." Pediatric pulmonology 36.6 (2003): 514-521

Boutelle, Kerri, et al. "Weight control behaviors among obese, overweight, and nonoverweight adolescents." Journal of Pediatric Psychology 27.6 (2002): 531-540.

Foster, Gary D., et al. "Primary care physicians' attitudes about obesity and its treatment." Obesity Research 11.10 (2012): 1168-1177.

Stunkard, Albert J., and Thomas A. Wadden. "Psychological aspects of severe obesity." The American journal of clinical nutrition 55.2 (1992): 524S-532S.

MacLean, Lynne, et al. "Obesity, stigma and public health planning." Health Promotion International 24.1 (2009): 88-93.

Puhl, Rebecca M., and Chelsea A. Heuer. "The stigma of obesity: a review and update." Obesity 17.5 (2012): 941-964.

Wear, Delese, et al. "Making fun of patients: medical students' perceptions and use of derogatory and cynical humor in clinical settings." Academic Medicine81.5 (2006): 454-462.

Amy, Nancy K., et al. "Barriers to routine gynecological cancer screening for White and African-American obese women." International Journal of Obesity30.1 (2005): 147-155.

Szwarc, Sandy. "Putting facts over fears: examining childhood anti-obesity initiatives." International Quarterly of Community Health Education 23.2 (2004): 97-116.

Burgard, Debora, and Pat Lyons. "Alternatives in obesity treatment: Focusing on health for fat women." Feminist perspectives on eating disorders (1994): 212-230.

National Task Force on the Prevention and Treatment of Obesity; "Medical Care for Obese Patients: Advice for Health Care Professionals
Am Fam Physician. 2002 Jan 1;65(1):81-88.

Wadden, Thomas A., and Elizabeth Didie. "What's in a name? Patients' preferred terms for describing obesity." Obesity 11.9 (2003): 1140-1146.

Chapter 3 References

Kalm, Leah M., and Richard D. Semba. "They starved so that others be better fed: remembering Ancel Keys and the Minnesota experiment." The Journal of nutrition 135.6 (2005): 1347-1352.

http://mbbnet.umn.edu/hoff/hoff_ak.html describes the work of Ancel Keys

Leibel, Rudolph L., and Jules Hirsch. "Diminished energy requirements in reduced-obese patients." Metabolism 33.2 (1984): 164-170.

Leibel, Rudolph L., Michael Rosenbaum, and Jules Hirsch. "Changes in energy expenditure resulting from altered body weight." New England Journal of Medicine 332.10 (1995): 621-628.

Bouchard, Claude, et al. "The response to long-term overfeeding in identical twins." New England Journal of Medicine 322.21 (1990): 1477-1482.

Goran, Michael I. "Genetic influences on human energy expenditure and substrate utilization." Behavior genetics 27.4 (1997): 389-399.

Sims, ETHAN AH, EDWARD S. Horton, and LESTER B. Salans. "Inducible metabolic abnormalities during development of obesity." Annual review of medicine 22.1 (1971): 235-248.

SIMS, ETHAN AH, and EDWARD S. HORTON. "Endocrine and metabolic adaptation to obesity and starvation." The American journal of clinical nutrition21.12 (1968): 1455-1470.

Salans, Lester B., Samuel W. Cushman, and Rodger E. Weismann. "Studies of human adipose tissue Adipose cell size and number in nonobese and obese patients." Journal of clinical investigation 52.4 (1973): 929.

Weyer, Christian, et al. "Energy expenditure, fat oxidation, and body weight regulation: a study of metabolic adaptation to long-term weight change." Journal of Clinical Endocrinology & Metabolism 85.3 (2000): 1087-1094.

Thomas, Olivia, et al. "Industry funding and the reporting quality of large long-term weight loss trials." International Journal of Obesity 32.10 (2008): 1531-1536.

Blundell, John E., and Angela Gillett. "Control of food intake in the obese."Obesity research 9.S11 (2001): 263S-270S.

Blundell, John E. "What foods do people habitually eat? A dilemma for nutrition, an enigma for psychology." The American journal of clinical nutrition 71.1 (2000): 3-5.

Salans, Lester B., Samuel W. Cushman, and Rodger E. Weismann. "Studies of human adipose tissue Adipose cell size and number in nonobese and obese patients." Journal of clinical investigation 52.4 (1973): 929.

Tsai, Adam Gilden, and Thomas A. Wadden. "Systematic review: an evaluation of major commercial weight loss programs in the United States." Annals of Internal Medicine 142.1 (2005): 56-66.

Caplan, W. I. L. L. I. A. M., JILL D. Bowman, and NICOLAS P. Pronk. "Weight-loss outcomes: a systematic review and meta-analysis of weight-loss clinical trials with a minimum 1-year follow-up." J Am Diet Assoc 107 (2007): 1755-1767.

Thorsdottir, I., et al. "Randomized trial of weight-loss-diets for young adults varying in fish and fish oil content." International journal of obesity 31.10 (2007): 1560-1566.

Ramel, Alfons, Margret Thora Jonsdottir, and Inga Thorsdottir. "Consumption of cod and weight loss in young overweight and obese adults on an energy reduced diet for 8-weeks." Nutrition, metabolism and cardiovascular diseases19.10 (2009): 690-696.

Scientific Advisory Committee on Nutrition "Advice on fish consumption: Benefits and Risks" published for the Food Standards Agency 2004.

Ash, Susan, et al. "Effect of intensive dietetic interventions on weight and glycaemic control in overweight men with Type II diabetes: a randomised trial."International journal of obesity 27.7 (2003): 797-802.

Stubbs, R. James, et al. "Covert manipulation of dietary fat and energy density: effect on substrate flux and food intake in men eating ad libitum." The American journal of clinical nutrition 62.2 (1995): 316-329.

Stubbs, R. J., et al. "Covert manipulation of the ratio of dietary fat to carbohydrate and energy density: effect on food intake and energy balance in free-living men eating ad libitum." The American journal of clinical nutrition 62.2 (1995): 330-337.

Stubbs, R. J., et al. "How covert are covertly manipulated diets?." International journal of obesity and related metabolic disorders: journal of the International Association for the Study of Obesity 25.4 (2001): 567.

de Souza, Russell J., et al. "Effects of 4 weight-loss diets differing in fat, protein, and carbohydrate on fat mass, lean mass, visceral adipose tissue, and hepatic fat: results from the POUNDS LOST trial." The American journal of clinical nutrition 95.3 (2012): 614-625.

Sacks, Frank M., et al. "Comparison of weight-loss diets with different compositions of fat, protein, and carbohydrates." New England Journal of Medicine 360.9 (2009): 859-873.

Lagiou, Pagona, et al. "Low carbohydrate-high protein diet and incidence of cardiovascular diseases in Swedish women: prospective cohort study." BMJ: British Medical Journal 344 (2012).

Floegel, Anna, and Tobias Pischon. "Low carbohydrate-high protein diets."BMJ: British Medical Journal 344 (2012).

Floegel, Anna, and Tobias Pischon. "Editorial authors' reply to Freedhoff." BMJ: British Medical Journal 345 (2012).

Katan, Martijn B. "Weight-loss diets for the prevention and treatment of obesity." New England Journal of Medicine 360.9 (2009): 923-925.

Anson, R. Michael, et al. "Intermittent fasting dissociates beneficial effects of dietary restriction on glucose metabolism and neuronal resistance to injury from calorie intake." Proceedings of the National Academy of Sciences 100.10 (2003): 6216-6220.

Masoro, Edward J. "Caloric restriction and aging: an update." Experimental gerontology 35.3 (2000): 299-305.

Weindruch, Richard, and Rajindar S. Sohal. "Caloric intake and aging." The New England journal of medicine 337.14 (1997): 986.

Alirezaei, Mehrdad, et al. "Short-term fasting induces profound neuronal autophagy." Autophagy 6.6 (2010): 702-710.

Fontana, Luigi, Linda Partridge, and Valter D. Longo. "Extending healthy life span—from yeast to humans." science 328.5976 (2010): 321-326.

Heilbronn, Leonie K., et al. "Alternate-day fasting in nonobese subjects: effects on body weight, body composition, and energy metabolism." The American journal of clinical nutrition 81.1 (2005): 69-73.

Harvie, Michelle N., et al. "The effects of intermittent or continuous energy restriction on weight loss and metabolic disease risk markers: a randomized trial in young overweight women." International Journal of Obesity 35.5 (2010): 714-727.

M N Harvie "Intermittent low carbohydrate diets more successful than standard dieting; possible intervention for breast cancer prevention" presentation of poster at the CTRCAACR San Antonio Breast Cancer Symposium. www.aacr.org/home/public--media/aacr-press-releases.aspx?d=2649

Sandholt, C. H., T. Hansen, and O. Pedersen. "Beyond the fourth wave of genome-wide obesity association studies." Nutrition & diabetes 2.7 (2012): e37.

Varady, Krista A., et al. "Short-term modified alternate-day fasting: a novel dietary strategy for weight loss and cardioprotection in obese adults." The American journal of clinical nutrition 90.5 (2009): 1138-1143.

Varady, Krista A., and Marc K. Hellerstein. "Alternate-day fasting and chronic disease prevention: a review of human and animal trials." The American journal of clinical nutrition 86.1 (2007): 7-13.

Johnson, James B., et al. "Alternate day calorie restriction improves clinical findings and reduces markers of oxidative stress and inflammation in overweight adults with moderate asthma." Free Radical Biology and Medicine 42.5 (2007): 665-674.

Johnson, James B., Donald R. Laub, and Sujit John. "The effect on health of alternate day calorie restriction: eating less and more than needed on alternate days prolongs life." Medical hypotheses 67.2 (2006): 209-211.

Stote, Kim S., et al. "A controlled trial of reduced meal frequency without caloric restriction in healthy, normal-weight, middle-aged adults." The American journal of clinical nutrition 85.4 (2007): 981-988.

Johnstone, A. M. "Fasting–the ultimate diet?." obesity reviews 8.3 (2007): 211-222.

Stewart, W. K., and Laura W. Fleming. "Features of a successful therapeutic fast of 382 days' duration." Postgraduate medical journal 49.569 (1973): 203-209.

Hu, Frank B., et al. "Trends in the incidence of coronary heart disease and changes in diet and lifestyle in women." New England Journal of Medicine 343.8 (2000): 530-537.

Ludwig, David S., et al. "High glycemic index foods, overeating, and obesity."Pediatrics 103.3 (1999): e26-e26.

Hunt, J. N., and D. F. Stubbs. "The volume and energy content of meals as determinants of gastric emptying." The Journal of physiology 245.1 (1975): 209-225.

Hunt, J. N., R. Cash, and P. Newland. "Energy density of food, gastric emptying, and obesity." Lancet 2.7941 (1975): 905.

Leathwood, Peter, and Patricia Pollet. "Effects of slow release carbohydrates in the form of bean flakes on the evolution of hunger and satiety in man." Appetite10.1 (1988): 1-11.

Holt, S. H., Miller JC Brand, and P. Petocz. "Interrelationships among postprandial satiety, glucose and insulin responses and changes in subsequent food intake." European journal of clinical nutrition 50.12 (1996): 788.

Raben, A2 "Should obese patients be counselled to follow a low - glycaemic index diet? No." Obesity reviews 3.4 (2002): 245-256

Atkinson, Fiona S., Kaye Foster-Powell, and Jennie C. Brand-Miller. "International tables of glycemic index and glycemic load values: 2008."Diabetes Care 31.12 (2008): 2281-2283.

Tsai, Adam Gilden and Thomas A. Wadden "The evolution of very low calorie diets: an update and meta-analysis" Obesity 14.8 (2006): 1283-1293

http://www.nytimes.com/1988/11/24/us/health-nutrition-diet-that-made-oprah-winfrey-slim-demands-discipline.html

Gardner, Christopher D., et al. "Comparison of the Atkins, Zone, Ornish, and LEARN diets for change in weight and related risk factors among overweight premenopausal women." JAMA: the journal of the American Medical Association 297.9 (2007): 969-977.

Dansinger, Michael L., et al. "Comparison of the Atkins, Ornish, Weight Watchers, and Zone diets for weight loss and heart disease risk reduction."JAMA: the journal of the American Medical Association 293.1 (2005): 43-53.

Lagiou, Pagona, et al. "Low carbohydrate-high protein diet and incidence of cardiovascular diseases in Swedish women: prospective cohort study." BMJ: British Medical Journal 344 (2012).

Ashley, Judith M., et al. "Meal replacements in weight intervention." Obesity research 9.S11 (2001): 312S-320S.

Heshka, Stanley, et al. "Weight loss with self-help compared with a structured commercial program." JAMA: the journal of the American Medical Association289.14 (2003): 1792-1798.

Ditschuneit, Herwig H and Marion Flechtner-Mors. "Value of Structured Meals for Weght Management; Risk Factors and Long-Term Weight Maintenance. "Obesity Reserarch 9.S11 (2001): 284S-289S.

Noakes, Manny, et al. "Meal replacements are as effective as structured weight-loss diets for treating obesity in adults with features of metabolic syndrome." The Journal of nutrition 134.8 (2004): 1894-1899.

Quinn Rothacker, Dana. "Five-year self-management of weight using meal replacements: comparison with matched controls in rural Wisconsin." Nutrition16.5 (2000): 344-348.

Heymsfield, S. B., et al. "Weight management using a meal replacement strategy: meta and pooling analysis from six studies." International journal of obesity 27.5 (2003): 537-549.

Wing, Rena R., and Robert W. Jeffery. "Food provision as a strategy to

226

promote weight loss." Obesity research 9.S11 (2001): 271S-275S.

Rock, Cheryl L., et al. "Randomized trial of a multifaceted commercial weight loss program." Obesity 15.4 (2007): 939-949.

Rock, Cheryl L., et al. "Effect of a free prepared meal and incentivized weight loss program on weight loss and weight loss maintenance in obese and overweight women." JAMA: The Journal of the American Medical Association304.16 (2010): 1803-1810.

Koh-Banerjee, Pauline, and Eric B. Rimm. "Whole grain consumption and weight gain: a review of the epidemiological evidence, potential mechanisms and opportunities for future research." PROCEEDINGS-NUTRITION SOCIETY OF LONDON. Vol. 62. No. 1. CABI Publishing; 1999, 2003.

Williams, Peter G., Sara J. Grafenauer, and Jane E. O'Shea. "Cereal grains, legumes, and weight management: a comprehensive review of the scientific evidence." Nutrition reviews 66.4 (2008): 171-182.

Schulz, Mandy, et al. "Food groups as predictors for short-term weight changes in men and women of the EPIC-Potsdam cohort." The Journal of nutrition 132.6 (2002): 1335-1340.

Abete, Itziar, et al. "Obesity and the metabolic syndrome: role of different dietary macronutrient distribution patterns and specific nutritional components on weight loss and maintenance." Nutrition reviews 68.4 (2010): 214-231.

Yanovski, Jack A., et al. "Effects of Calcium Supplementation on Body Weight and Adiposity in Overweight and Obese AdultsA Randomized Trial." Annals of internal medicine 150.12 (2009): 821-829.

Ard, Jamy D., et al. "The effect of the PREMIER interventions on insulin sensitivity." Diabetes Care 27.2 (2004): 340-347.

Hill, Alison M., et al. "Can EGCG reduce abdominal fat in obese subjects?."Journal of the American College of Nutrition 26.4 (2007): 396S-402S.

Maki, Kevin C., et al. "Green tea catechin consumption enhances exercise-induced abdominal fat loss in overweight and obese adults." The Journal of nutrition 139.2 (2009): 264-270.

Phung, Olivia J., et al. "Effect of green tea catechins with or without caffeine on anthropometric measures: a systematic review and meta-analysis." The American journal of clinical nutrition 91.1 (2010): 73-81.

Hursel, R., W. Viechtbauer, and M. S. Westerterp-Plantenga. "The effects of green tea on weight loss and weight maintenance: a meta-analysis."International journal of obesity 33.9 (2009): 956-961.

Crujeiras, Ana B., et al. "A role for fruit content in energy-restricted diets in improving antioxidant status in obese women during weight loss." Nutrition 22.6 (2006): 593-599.

Rolls, Barbara J., and Elizabeth A. Bell. "Dietary approaches to the treatment of obesity." Medical Clinics of North America 84.2 (2000): 401-418.

Rolls, Barbara J., Adam Drewnowski, and Jenny H. Ledikwe. "Changing the energy density of the diet as a strategy for weight management." Journal of the American Dietetic Association 105.5 (2005): 98-103.

Abete, Itziar, et al. "Obesity and the metabolic syndrome: role of different dietary macronutrient distribution patterns and specific nutritional components on weight loss and maintenance." Nutrition reviews 68.4 (2010): 214-231.

Lowe, Michael R. "Self-Regulation of Energy Intake in the Prevention and Treatment of Obesity: Is It Feasible?." OBESITY RESEARCH 11 (2003): 45S.

Morgan, Philip J et al "12-month outcomes and process evaluation of the SHED-IT RCT an internet-based weight loss program targeting men" Obesity 19.1 (2011): 142-151

McConnon, Áine, et al. "The Internet for weight control in an obese sample: results of a randomised controlled trial." BMC health services research 7.1 (2007): 206.

Johnson, Fiona, and Jane Wardle. "The association between weight loss and engagement with a web-based food and exercise diary in a commercial weight loss programme: a retrospective analysis." Int J Behav Nutr Phys Act 8 (2011): 83.

Harvey-Berino, Jean, et al. "Internet delivered behavioral obesity treatment."Preventive medicine 51.2 (2010): 123-128.

Brouwer, Wendy, et al. "Which intervention characteristics are related to more exposure to internet-delivered healthy lifestyle promotion interventions? A systematic review." Journal of medical Internet research 13.1 (2011).

Wantland, Dean J., et al. "The effectiveness of Web-based vs. non-Web-based interventions: a meta-analysis of behavioral change outcomes." Journal of medical Internet research 6.4 (2004).

Saris, W. H., et al. "Randomized controlled trial of changes in dietary carbohydrate/fat ratio and simple vs complex carbohydrates on body weight and blood lipids: the CARMEN study." International journal of obesity 24.10 (2000): 1310-1318.

Urbszat, Dax, C. Peter Herman, and Janet Polivy. "Eat, drink, and be merry, for tomorrow we diet: effects of anticipated deprivation on food intake in restrained and unrestrained eaters." Journal of Abnormal Psychology 111.2 (2002): 396-401.

Hill, Andrew J. "Does dieting make you fat?." British Journal of Nutrition 92.S1 (2004): S15-S18.

Patton, G. C., et al. "Onset of adolescent eating disorders: population based cohort study over 3 years." BMJ: British Medical Journal 318.7186 (1999): 765.

Chapter 4 References

http://www.sportengland.org/research/active_people_survey/active_people_survey_51.aspx statistics about sport participation

Levine, James A., et al. "Non-Exercise Activity Thermogenesis The Crouching Tiger Hidden Dragon of Societal Weight Gain." Arteriosclerosis, Thrombosis, and Vascular Biology 26.4 (2006): 729-736.

Levine, James A., et al. "The role of free-living daily walking in human weight gain and obesity." Diabetes 57.3 (2008): 548-554.

Lanningham-Foster, Lorraine, Lana J. Nysse, and James A. Levine. "Labor saved, calories lost: the energetic impact of domestic labor-saving devices."Obesity 11.10 (2003): 1178-1181.

Levine, James A., et al. "Interindividual variation in posture allocation: possible role in human obesity." Science 307.5709 (2005): 584-586.

Stubbs, R. James, et al. "The effect of graded levels of exercise on energy intake and balance in free-living men, consuming their normal diet." European journal of clinical nutrition 56 (2002): 129-140.

Stubbs, R. James, et al. "The effect of graded levels of exercise on energy intake and balance in free-living women." International journal of obesity and related metabolic disorders: journal of the International Association for the Study of Obesity 26.6 (2002): 866-869.

Pomerleau, Marjorie, et al. "Effects of exercise intensity on food intake and appetite in women." The American journal of clinical nutrition 80.5 (2004): 1230-1236.

Hagobian, Todd A., et al. "Effects of exercise on energy-regulating hormones and appetite in men and women." American Journal of Physiology-Regulatory, Integrative and Comparative Physiology 296.2 (2009): R233-R

Finlayson, Graham, et al. "Acute compensatory eating following exercise is associated with implicit hedonic wanting for food." Physiology & behavior 97.1 (2009): 62-67.

Finlayson, Graham, et al. "Low fat loss response after medium-term supervised exercise in obese is associated with exercise-induced increase in food reward."Journal of obesity 2011 (2010).

King, Neil A., et al. "Individual variability following 12 weeks of supervised exercise: identification and characterization of compensation for exercise-induced weight loss." International Journal of Obesity 32.1 (2007): 177-184.

Lluch, A., N. A. King, and J. E. Blundell. "Exercise in dietary restrained women: no effect on energy intake but change in hedonic ratings." European journal of clinical nutrition 52.4 (1998): 30

King, Neil A., et al. "Dual-process action of exercise on appetite control: increase in orexigenic drive but improvement in meal-induced satiety." The American journal of clinical nutrition 90.4 (2009): 921-927.

Long, S. J., K. Hart, and L. M. Morgan. "The ability of habitual exercise to influence appetite and food intake in response to high-and low-energy preloads in man." British Journal of Nutrition 87.5 (2002): 517-523

Fredericson, Michael, and Anuruddh K. Misra. "Epidemiology and aetiology of marathon running injuries." Sports Medicine 37.4-5 (2007): 437-439.

Stubbe, Janine H., et al. "Genetic influences on exercise participation in 37.051 twin pairs from seven countries." PLoS One 1.1 (2006): e22.

Boomsma, Dorret, Andreas Busjahn, and Leena Peltonen. "Classical twin studies and beyond." Nature reviews genetics 3.11 (2002): 872-882.

Vink, Jacqueline M., et al. "Variance components models for physical activity with age as modifier: a comparative twin study in seven countries." Twin Research and Human Genetics 14.01 (2011): 25-34.

Stubbe, Janine H., and Eco JC de Geus. "Genetics of exercise behavior."Handbook of behavior genetics. Springer New York, 2009. 343-358.

Tergerson, Jennifer L., and Keith A. King. "Do perceived cues, benefits, and barriers to physical activity differ between male and female adolescents?."Journal of school health 72.9 (2002): 374-380.

Bouchard, Claude, and A. Tremblay. "Genetic effects in human energy expenditure components." International journal of obesity 14 (1990): 49.

De Moor, M. H. M., et al. "Regular exercise, anxiety, depression and personality: a population-based study." Preventive medicine 42.4 (2006): 273-279.

De Moor, Marleen HM, et al. "Testing causality in the association between regular exercise and symptoms of anxiety and depression." Archives of General Psychiatry 65.8 (2008): 897.

Lightfoot, J. Timothy. "Current understanding of the genetic basis for physical activity." The Journal of nutrition 141.3 (2011): 526-530.

Joosen, Annemiek MCP, et al. "Genetic analysis of physical activity in twins."The American journal of clinical nutrition 82.6 (2005): 1253-1259.

Thorburn, A. W., and J. Proietto. "Biological determinants of spontaneous physical activity." Obesity Reviews 1.2 (2000): 87-94.

http://www.telegraph.co.uk/culture/tvandradio/bbc/9202922/BBC-in-new-sexism-row-after-gender-pay-gap-revealed.html statistics on male and female managers in the BBC

Moore, Lynn L., et al. "Influence of parents' physical activity levels on activity levels of young children." The Journal of pediatrics 118.2 (1991): 215-219.

Mallam, Katie M., et al. "Contribution of timetabled physical education to total physical activity in primary school children: cross sectional study." Bmj327.7415 (2003): 592-593.

Goran, MICHAEL I., and ERIC T. Poehlman. "Endurance training does not enhance total energy expenditure in healthy elderly persons." American Journal of Physiology-Endocrinology And Metabolism 263.5 (1992): E950-E957.

Thorburn, A. W., and J. Proietto. "Biological determinants of spontaneous physical activity." Obesity Reviews 1.2 (2000): 87-94.

King, Neil A., et al. "Metabolic and behavioral compensatory responses to exercise interventions: barriers to weight loss." Obesity 15.6 (2007): 1373-1383.

Meijer, G. A. L., et al. "The effect of a 5-month endurance-training programme on physical activity: evidence for a sex-difference in the metabolic response to exercise." European journal of applied physiology and occupational physiology62.1 (1991): 11-17.

Frey-Hewitt, B., et al. "The effect of weight loss by dieting or exercise on resting metabolic rate in overweight men." International journal of obesity 14.4 (1990): 327.

King, N. A., et al. "Effects of short-term exercise on appetite responses in unrestrained females." European journal of clinical nutrition 50.10 (1996): 663-667.

Donnelly, Joseph E., et al. "Effects of a 16-month randomized controlled exercise trial on body weight and composition in young, overweight men and women: the Midwest Exercise Trial." Archives of Internal Medicine 163.11 (2003): 1343.

Plasqui Guy et al "Measuring free-living energy expenditure and physical activity with triaxial accelerometry" Obesity Research 13.8 (2005): 1363-1369

Weinsier, Roland L., et al. "Free-living activity energy expenditure in women successful and unsuccessful at maintaining a normal body weight." The American journal of clinical nutrition 75.3 (2002): 499-504.

Slentz, Cris A., et al. "Effects of the amount of exercise on body weight, body composition, and measures of central obesity: STRRIDE--a randomized controlled study." Archives of Internal Medicine 164.1 (2004): 31.

Hill, James O., et al. "Effects of exercise and food restriction on body composition and metabolic rate in obese women." The American journal of clinical nutrition 46.4 (1987): 622-630.

Curioni, C. C., and P. M. Lourenco. "Long-term weight loss after diet and exercise: a systematic review." International Journal of Obesity 29.10 (2005): 1168-1174.

Miller, Wayne C., D. M. Koceja, and E. J. Hamilton. "A meta-analysis of the past 25 years of weight loss research using diet, exercise or diet plus exercise intervention." International journal of obesity 21.10 (1997): 941-947.

Blundell, John E., et al. "Cross talk between physical activity and appetite control: does physical activity stimulate appetite?." Proceedings of the Nutrition Society 62.03 (2003): 651-661.

Chapter 5 References

http://www.dailymail.co.uk/femail/article-1035279/From-fat-fit--fat-The-celebrity-workout-DVDs-didnt-quite-work-.html

Wing, Rena R., and Suzanne Phelan. "Long-term weight loss maintenance."The American journal of clinical nutrition 82.1 (2005): 222S-225S.

Wing, Rena R., and James O. Hill. "Successful weight loss maintenance."Annual review of nutrition 21.1 (2001): 323-341.

Kruger, Judy, Heidi M. Blanck, and Cathleen Gillespie. "Dietary and physical activity behaviors among adults successful at weight loss maintenance."International Journal of Behavioral Nutrition and Physical Activity 3.1 (2006): 17.

Ogden, Lorraine G., et al. "Cluster analysis of the national weight control registry to identify distinct subgroups maintaining successful weight loss."Obesity (2012).

Phelan, Suzanne, et al. "Holiday weight management by successful weight losers and normal weight individuals." Kinesiology (2008): 22.

Frazao, Elizabeth. "America's eating habits: changes and consequences."Agriculture Information Bulletin-United States Department of Agriculture 750 (1999).

Kayman, Susan, William Bruvold, and Judith S. Stern. "Maintenance and relapse after weight loss in women: behavioral aspects." The American journal of clinical nutrition 52.5 (1990): 800-807.

Elfhag, K., and S. Rössner. "Who succeeds in maintaining weight loss? A conceptual review of factors associated with weight loss maintenance and weight regain." Obesity reviews 6.1 (2005): 67-85.

Byrne, Susan M., Zafra Cooper, and Christopher G. Fairburn. "Psychological predictors of weight regain in obesity." Behaviour research and therapy 42.11 (2004): 1341-1356.

Byrne, S., Z. Cooper, and C. Fairburn. "Weight maintenance and relapse in obesity: a qualitative study." International journal of obesity 27.8 (2003): 955-962.

Wing, Rena R., et al. "A self-regulation program for maintenance of weight loss." New England Journal of Medicine 355.15 (2006): 1563-1571.

Stuart, RICHARD B., and Kenneth Guire. "Some correlates of the maintenance of weight lost through behavior modification." International journal of obesity 2.2 (1978): 225.

Epstein, Leonard H., and Patricia A. Cluss. "A behavioral medicine perspective on adherence to long-term medical regimens." Journal of consulting and clinical psychology 50.6 (1982): 950.

Chapter 6 References

Muller, Ulrich, and Allan Mazur. "Facial dominance in Homo sapiens as honest signaling of male quality." Behavioral Ecology 8.5 (1997): 569-579.

Dion, Karen K. "Physical attractiveness and evaluation of children's transgressions." Journal of Personality and Social Psychology 24.2 (1972): 207.

Benson, Peter L., Stuart A. Karabenick, and Richard M. Lerner. "Pretty pleases: The effects of physical attractiveness, race, and sex on receiving help." Journal of Experimental Social Psychology 12.5 (1976): 409-415.

Clayson, Dennis E., and Michael L. Klassen. "Perception of attractiveness by obesity and hair color." Perceptual and Motor Skills 68.1 (1989): 199-202.

Klassen, Michael L., "The cognitive basis of social judgment;the role of stereotypical beliefs in the processing of information about obese and thin people" Kansas State university 1987

Roehling, Mark V., Patricia V. Roehling, and L. Maureen Odland. "Investigating the Validity of Stereotypes About Overweight Employees The Relationship Between Body Weight and Normal Personality Traits." Group & Organization Management 33.4 (2008): 392-424.

Brummett, Beverly H., et al. "Personality as a predictor of dietary quality in spouses during midlife." Behavioral Medicine 34.1 (2008): 5-10.

Rothblum, Esther D., et al. "The relationship between obesity, employment discrimination, and employment-related victimization." Journal of Vocational Behavior 37.3 (1990): 251-266.

Karris, Lambros. "Prejudice against obese renters." The Journal of Social Psychology (1977).

Puhl, Rebecca M., and Kelly D. Brownell. "Confronting and coping with weight stigma: an investigation of overweight and obese adults." Obesity 14.10 (2012): 1802-1815.

Puhl, Rebecca M., and Chelsea A. Heuer. "The stigma of obesity: a review and update." Obesity 17.5 (2012): 941-964.

Crandall, Christian S. "Prejudice against fat people: ideology and self-interest."Journal of personality and social psychology 66.5 (1994): 882.

Hebl, Michelle R., and Laura M. Mannix. "The weight of obesity in evaluating others: A mere proximity effect." Personality and Social Psychology Bulletin29.1 (2003): 28-38.

Pingitore, Regina, et al. "Bias against overweight job applicants in a simulated employment interview." Journal of Applied Psychology; Journal of Applied Psychology 79.6 (1994): 909.

Swami, Viren, et al. "An investigation of weight bias against women and its associations with individual difference factors." Body image 7.3 (2010): 194-199.

Puhl, Rebecca M., and Chelsea A. Heuer. "The stigma of obesity: a review and update." Obesity 17.5 (2012): 941-964.

Crandall, Christian and Monica Biernat. "The Ideology of Anti-Fat Attitudes 1" Journal of Applied Social psychology 20.3 (2006): 227-243

Puhl, Rebecca M., et al. "Weight stigmatization and bias reduction: perspectives of overweight and obese adults." Health Education Research 23.2 (2008): 347-358.

King, Eden B., et al. "The stigma of obesity in customer service: a mechanism for remediation and bottom-line consequences of interpersonal discrimination."Journal of Applied Psychology 91.3 (2006): 579.

Hebl, Michelle R., and Todd F. Heatherton. "The stigma of obesity in women: The difference is black and white." Personality and Social Psychology Bulletin24 (1998): 417-426.

Puhl, Rebecca, and Kelly D. Brownell. "Bias, discrimination, and obesity."Obesity research 9.12 (2012): 788-805.

Crandall, Christian S. "Do heavy-weight students have more difficulty paying for college?" Personality and Social Psychology Bulletin 17.6 (1991):

606-611.

Crandall, Christian S. "Do parents discriminate against their heavyweight daughters?." Personality and Social Psychology Bulletin 21.7 (1995): 724-735.

Karnehed, Nina, et al. "Obesity and attained education: cohort study of more than 700,000 Swedish men." Obesity 14.8 (2012): 1421-1428.

Hamermesh, Daniel S., and Jeff E. Biddle. Beauty and the labor market. No. w4518. National Bureau of Economic Research, 1993.

Rothblum, Esther D., et al. "The relationship between obesity, employment discrimination, and employment-related victimization." Journal of Vocational Behavior 37.3 (1990): 251-266.

Hebl, Michelle R., and Laura M. Mannix. "The weight of obesity in evaluating others: A mere proximity effect." Personality and Social Psychology Bulletin29.1 (2003): 28-38.

Pingitore, Regina, et al. "Bias against overweight job applicants in a simulated employment interview." Journal of Applied Psychology; Journal of Applied Psychology 79.6 (1994): 909.

Melville, D. Scott, and Bradley J. Cardinal. "Are Overweight Physical Educators At a Disadvantage in the Labor Market? A Random Survey of Hiring Personnel."Physical Educator 54.4 (1997): 216-21.

Cawley, John, and Sheldon Danziger. Obesity as a barrier to the transition from welfare to work. No. w10508. National Bureau of Economic Research, 2004.

Carr, Deborah, and Michael A. Friedman. "Is obesity stigmatizing? Body weight, perceived discrimination, and psychological well-being in the United States." Journal of Health and Social Behavior 46.3 (2005): 244-259.

Sargent, James D., and David G. Blanchflower. "Obesity and stature in adolescence and earnings in young adulthood: analysis of a British birth cohort." Archives of Pediatrics & Adolescent Medicine 148.7 (1994): 681

Morris, Stephen. "Body mass index and occupational attainment." Journal of Health Economics 25.2 (2006): 347-364.

Puhl, Rebecca M., and Chelsea A. Heuer. "The stigma of obesity: a review and update." Obesity 17.5 (2012): 941-964.

Averett, Susan, and Sanders Korenman. The economic reality of the beauty myth. No. w4521. National Bureau of Economic Research, 1993.

Gortmaker, Steven L., et al. "Social and economic consequences of overweight in adolescence and young adulthood." New England journal of medicine 329.14 (1993): 1008-1012.

Sarlio-Lähteenkorva, Sirpa, Karri Silventoinen, and Eero Lahelma. "Relative weight and income at different levels of socioeconomic status." Journal Information 94.3 (2004).

Kortt, Michael, and Andrew Leigh. "Does Size Matter in Australia?*." Economic Record 86.272 (2009): 71-83.

http://www.personneltoday.com/articles/25/10/2005/32213/obesity-research-fattism-is-the-last-bastion-of-employee.htm#.UTSmTqJvXjs

Bellizzi, Joseph A., and Ronald W. Hasty. "Territory assignment decisions and supervising unethical selling behavior: the effects of obesity and gender as moderated by job-related factors." The Journal of Personal Selling and Sales Management (1998): 35-49.

Bordieri, James E., David E. Drehmer, and Darrell W. Taylor. "Work life for employees with disabilities: Recommendations for promotion." Rehabilitation Counseling Bulletin (1997).

Roehling, Patricia V., et al. "Weight discrimination and the glass ceiling effect among top US CEOs." Equal Opportunities International 28.2 (2009): 179-196.

Ministerial Task Force for Health, Safety and Productivity and the Cabinet Office (2004) Managing sickness absence in the public sector. London: Health and Safety Executive

Rothblum, Esther D., et al. "The relationship between obesity, employment discrimination, and employment-related victimization." Journal of Vocational Behavior 37.3 (1990): 251-266.

Roehling Mark V "Weight-based discrimination in employment: psychological and legal aspects." Personnel Psychology 52.4 (2006): 969-1016

Gates Donna M, EdD, RN, FAAN JOEM Obesity and Presenteeism: The Impact of Body Mass Index on Workplace Productivity •Volume 50, Number 1, January 2008

Ferrie, Jane E., et al. "BMI, obesity, and sickness absence in the Whitehall II study." Obesity 15.6 (2012): 1554-1564.

Moreau, M., et al. "Obesity, body fat distribution and incidence of sick leave in the Belgian workforce: the Belstress study." International journal of obesity28.4 (2004): 574-582.

Parkes, Katharine R. "Relative weight, smoking, and mental health as predictors of sickness and absence from work." Journal of Applied Psychology72.2 (1987): 275.

Tsai, Shan P., et al. "The impact of obesity on illness absence and productivity in an industrial population of petrochemical workers." Annals of epidemiology18.1 (2008): 8-14.

Goetzel, Ron Z., et al. "A Multi-Worksite Analysis of the Relationships among Body Mass Index, Medical Utilization and Worker Productivity." Journal of occupational and environmental medicine/American College of Occupational and Environmental Medicine 52.Suppl 1 (2010): S52.

Neovius, Kristian, et al. "Obesity status and sick leave: a systematic review."Obesity reviews 10.1 (2008): 17-27.

Roehling, Mark V. "Weight discrimination in the American workplace: ethical issues and analysis." Journal of Business Ethics 40.2 (2002): 177-189.

Klassen, Michael L., Dennis Clayson, and Cynthia R. Jasper. "Perceived effect of a salesperson's stigmatized appearance on store image: an experimental study of student's perceptions." International Review of Retail, Distribution and Consumer Research 6.2 (1996): 216-224.

Westover, Michael Lea, and Quint Randle. "Endorser weight and perceptions of brand attitude and intent to purchase." Journal of Promotion Management 15.1-2 (2009): 57-73.

http://www.nytimes.com/1985/05/08/nyregion/court-blocks-job-denials-for-obesity.html

Thomas, Daniel. "Fattism is the last bastion of employee discrimination."Personnel Today 25.4 (2005).

Post, Robert C., "Prejudicial Appearances: The Logic of American Antidiscrimination Law" (2000).Faculty Scholarship Series.Paper 192. http://digitalcommons.law.yale.edu/fss_papers/192

Kristen, Elizabeth. "Addressing the problem of weight discrimination in employment." California Law Review 90.1 (2002): 57-109.

Rhee, Jeannie Sclafani "Redressing for Success: The liability of Hooter's Restaurant for customer harassment of waitresses" Harv. Women's LJ 20(1997): 163-341

McKee, Keith, and Albert D. Smouse. "Clients' perceptions of counselor expertness, attractiveness, and trustworthiness: Initial impact of counselor status and weight." Journal of Counseling Psychology 30.3 (1983): 332.

Roehling, Mark V., Patricia V. Roehling, and Shaun Pichler. "The relationship between body weight and perceived weight-related employment discrimination: the role of sex and race." Journal of Vocational Behavior 71.2 (2007): 300-318.

Greenberg, Bradley S., et al. "Portrayals of overweight and obese individuals on commercial television." Journal Information 93.8 (2003).

Garner, David M., and Susan C. Wooley. "Confronting the failure of behavioral and dietary treatments for obesity." Clinical Psychology Review 11.6 (1991): 729-780.

Herbozo, Sylvia, et al. "Beauty and thinness messages in children's media: A content analysis." Eating Disorders 12.1 (2004): 21-34.

Fouts, Gregory, and Kimberley Vaughan. "Television situation comedies: Male weight, negative references, and audience reactions." Sex Roles 46.11 (2002): 439-442.

Fouts, Gregory, and Kimberley Burggraf. "Television situation comedies: Female weight, male negative comments, and audience reactions." Sex Roles42.9 (2000): 925-932.

Himes, Susan M., and J. Kevin Thompson. "Fat Stigmatization in Television Shows and Movies: A Content Analysis." (2007).

Moran, Lee "Passenger forced to stand 7 hours on US airways flight because of 400lb man sitting next to him" Daily Mail 24th November 2011

Puhl, Rebecca, and Kelly D. Brownell. "Bias, discrimination, and obesity."Obesity research 9.12 (2012): 788-805.

http://or.findacase.com/research/wfrmDocViewer.aspx/xq/fac.19950117_0 000003.DOR.htm/qx Sellick v Denny's

Pearce, Michelle J., Julie Boergers, and Mitchell J. Prinstein. "Adolescent obesity, overt and relational peer victimization, and romantic relationships."Obesity Research 10.5 (2012): 386-393.

Sheets, Virgil, and Kavita Ajmere. "Are romantic partners a source of college students' weight concern?." Eating behaviors 6.1 (2005): 1-9.

Chen, Eunice Y., and Molly Brown. "Obesity stigma in sexual relationships."Obesity Research 13.8 (2012): 1393-1397.

Puhl, Rebecca M., and Chelsea A. Heuer. "The stigma of obesity: a review and update." Obesity 17.5 (2012): 941-964.

Puhl, Rebecca, and Kelly D. Brownell. "Bias, discrimination, and obesity."Obesity research 9.12 (2012): 788-805.

Kimmel, Michael S., and Matthew Mahler. "Adolescent Masculinity, Homophobia, and Violence Random School Shootings, 1982-2001." American behavioral scientist 46.10 (2003): 1439-1458.

Davison, Kirsten Krahnstoever and Leann Lipps Birth "Predictors of Fat Stereotypes among 9 year old girls and their parents" Obesity Research 12.1 (2012): 86-94

Eisenberg, Marla E., Dianne Neumark-Sztainer, and Mary Story. "Associations of weight-based teasing and emotional well-being among adolescents."Archives of Pediatrics & Adolescent Medicine 157.8 (2003): 733.

Strauss, Richard S. "Childhood obesity and self-esteem." Pediatrics 105.1 (2000): e15-e15.

Pierce JW & Wardle J (1997): Cause and effect beliefs and self-esteem of overweight children. J. Child. Psychol. Psychiatry 38, 645–650.

Puhl RM, Brownell KD. Confronting and coping with weight stigma: An investigation of overweight and obese adults. Obesity 2006; 14: 1802–1815.

Tiggemann, Marika, and Tracy Anesbury. "Negative stereotyping of obesity in children: The role of controllability beliefs." Journal of Applied Social Psychology 30.9 (2006): 1977-1993.

Latner, Janet D., and Albert J. Stunkard. "Getting worse: the stigmatization of obese children." Obesity Research 11.3 (2012): 452-456.

Strauss, Richard S., and Harold A. Pollack. "Social marginalization of overweight children." Archives of Pediatrics & Adolescent Medicine 157.8 (2003): 746.

Reading Eagle/Reading Times Oct 2nd 1997 "British Teen takes Fatal Overdoes after "Fatty" Taunts"

Neumark-Sztainer, Dianne, Mary Story, and Tanya Harris. "Beliefs and attitudes about obesity among teachers and school health care providers working with adolescents." Journal of Nutrition Education 31.1 (1999): 3-9.

Puhl, Rebecca M., and Janet D. Latner. "Stigma, obesity, and the health of the nation's children." Psychological bulletin 133.4 (2007): 557.

Greenleaf, Christy, and Karen Weiller. "Perceptions of youth obesity among physical educators." Social Psychology of Education 8.4 (2005): 407-423.

Harrison, Kristen. "Television viewing, fat stereotyping, body shape standards, and eating disorder symptomatology in grade school children." Communication Research 27.5 (2000): 617-640.

Irving, Lori M. "Promoting size acceptance in elementary school children: the EDAP puppet program." Eating Disorders 8.3 (2000): 221-232.

Pierce, J. W. and Wardle, J. (1997) Cause and effect beliefs and self-esteem of overweight children. Journal of Child Psychology and Psychiatry and Allied Disciplines,38, 645–650.

Mellin, Alison E., et al. "Unhealthy behaviors and psychosocial difficulties among overweight adolescents: the potential impact of familial factors." Journal of Adolescent Health 31.2 (2002): 145-153.

Viner, Russell M., and Tim J. Cole. "Adult socioeconomic, educational, social, and psychological outcomes of childhood obesity: a national birth cohort study." bmj 330.7504 (2005): 1354.

Miller, Carol T., et al. "Compensating for stigma: Obese and nonobese women's reactions to being visible." Personality and Social Psychology Bulletin 21.10 (1995): 1093-1106.

Joanisse, Leanne, and Anthony Synnott. "Fighting back: Reactions and resistance to the stigma of obesity." Interpreting weight: The social management of fatness and thinness (1999): 49-70.

Puhl, Rebecca, and Kelly D. Brownell. "Ways of coping with obesity stigma: review and conceptual analysis." Eating Behaviors 4.1 (2003): 53-78.

Chapter 7 References

KOESLAG, JOHAN H. "The human biology of obesity, and its relevance to insurers." JOURNAL OF INSURANCE MEDICINE 22.1 (1990).

Snoek, Harriëtte M., Nienke Y. Sessink, and Rutger CME Engels. "Food choices of 4 to 6-year-old overweight and nonoverweight children while role-playing as adults." Journal of Family Psychology 24.6 (2010): 779.

Keskitalo, Kaisu, et al. "The Three-Factor Eating Questionnaire, body mass index, and responses to sweet and salty fatty foods: a twin study of genetic and environmental associations." The American journal of clinical nutrition 88.2 (2008): 263-271.

de Lauzon, Blandine, et al. "The Three-Factor Eating Questionnaire-R18 is able to distinguish among different eating patterns in a general population." The Journal of nutrition 134.9 (2004): 2372-2380.

Stice, Eric, Melissa Fisher, and Michael R. Lowe. "Are dietary restraint scales valid measures of acute dietary restriction? Unobtrusive observational data suggest not." Psychological assessment 16.1 (2004): 51.

Oshio, Atsushi. "Development and validation of the Dichotomous Thinking Inventory." Social Behavior and Personality: an international journal 37.6 (2009): 729-741.

Oshio, Atsushi, and Tatiana Meshkova. "Eating disorders, body image, and dichotomous thinking among Japanese and Russian college women." Health 4 (2012).

Koeslag, JOHAN H. "Human biology of obesity." S Afr J Contin Med Edu 8 (1990): 329-336.

Tsigos, Constantine, et al. "Management of obesity in adults: European clinical practice guidelines." Obesity facts 1.2 (2008): 106-116.

Darmon, Nicole, André Briend, and Adam Drewnowski. "Energy-dense diets are associated with lower diet costs: a community study of French adults." Public health nutrition 7.1 (2004): 21-28.

ABOUT THE AUTHOR

Alison Oates graduated in Medicine in Cardiff, in 1983. She worked in various specialties, including General Practice and Psychiatry, before taking on a role as a carer. She has written articles published in a journal for General Practitioners (family doctors).

ACKNOWLEDGEMENTS

Thanks to Janey, for her help in copy-editing. Also to Dorothy and David, for their encouragement in the writing of this book.

The website address that will be associated with this book is:

www.theweightissue.com

Printed in Great Britain
by Amazon.co.uk, Ltd.,
Marston Gate.